AO Manual of Fracture Management

Hans-Georg Dietz, Peter P Schmittenbecher, Theddy Slongo, Kaye E Wilkins

Elastic Stable Intramedullary Nailing (ESIN) in Children

AO Manual of Fracture Management

Hans-Georg Dietz, Peter P Schmittenbecher, Theddy Slongo, Kaye E Wilkins

Elastic Stable Intramedullary Nailing (ESIN) in Children

294 illustrations, 496 pictures and x-rays
30 step-by-step case descriptions

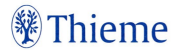

Design and layout: Sandro Isler, nougat GmbH, CH-4056 Basel
Illustrations: tadpole GmbH, CH-8048 Zürich

Library of Congress Cataloging-in-Publication Data is available from the publisher.

Hazards
Great care has been taken to maintain the accuracy of the information contained in this publication. However, the publisher, and/or the distributor, and/or the editors, and/or the authors cannot be held responsible for errors or any consequences arising from the use of the information contained in this publication. Contributions published under the name of individual authors are statements and opinions solely of said authors and not of the publisher, and/or the distributor, and/or the AO Group.
The products, procedures, and therapies described in this work are hazardous and are therefore only to be applied by certified and trained medical professionals in environments specially designed for such procedures. No suggested test or procedure should be carried out unless, in the user's professional judgment, its risk is justified. Whoever applies products, procedures, and therapies shown or described in this work will do this at their own risk. Because of rapid advances in the medical sciences, AO recommends that independent verification of diagnosis, therapies, drugs, dosages, and operation methods should be made before any action is taken.
Although all advertising material which may be inserted into the work is expected to conform to ethical (medical) standards, inclusion in this publication does not constitute a guarantee or endorsement by the publisher regarding quality or value of such product or of the claims made of it by its manufacturer.

Legal restrictions
This work was produced by AO Publishing, Davos, Switzerland. All rights reserved by AO Publishing. This publication, including all parts thereof, is legally protected by copyright. Any use, exploitation or commercialization outside the narrow limits set forth by copyright legislation and the restrictions on use laid out below, without the publisher's consent, is illegal and liable to prosecution. This applies in particular to photostat reproduction, copying, scanning or duplication of any kind, translation, preparation of microfilms, electronic data processing, and storage such as making this publication available on Intranet or Internet.
Some of the products, names, instruments, treatments, logos, designs, etc. referred to in this publication are also protected by patents and trademarks or by other intellectual property protection laws (eg, "AO", "ASIF", "AO/ASIF", "TRIANGLE/GLOBE Logo" are registered trademarks) even though specific reference to this fact is not always made in the text. Therefore, the appearance of a name, instrument, etc. without designation as proprietary is not to be construed as a representation by the publisher that it is in the public domain.
Restrictions on use: The rightful owner of an authorized copy of this work may use it for educational and research purposes only. Single images or illustrations may be copied for research or educational purposes only. The images or illustrations may not be altered in any way and need to carry the following statement of origin "Copyright by AO Publishing, Switzerland".

Copyright © 2006 by AO Publishing, Switzerland, Clavadelerstrasse 8, CH-7270 Davos Platz
Distribution by Georg Thieme Verlag, Rüdigerstrasse 14, DE-70469 Stuttgart and
Thieme New York, 333 Seventh Avenue, New York, NY 10001, USA

ISBN-10: 3-13-143331-0 (GTV)
ISBN-13: 978-3-13-143331-2 (GTV)
ISBN-10: 1-58890-485-7 (TNY)
ISBN-13: 978-1-58890-485-0 (TNY)

Contributors

Editors

Hans-Georg Dietz, MD
Professor of Pediatric Surgery
Ludwig-Maximilians-University
Munich
Dr. von Hauners Childrens Hospital
Department of Pediatric Surgery
Lindwurmstrasse 4
DE-80337 München

Peter P Schmittenbecher, MD
Ass. Professor of Pediatric Surgery
Clinical Center "Barmherzige Brüder"
Department of Pediatric Surgery
Steinmetzstrasse 1–3
DE-93049 Regensburg

Theddy Slongo, MD
Pediatric Trauma and Orthopedics
University Children's Hospital
Department of Pediatric Surgery
CH-3010 Bern

Kaye E Wilkins, DVM, MD
Professor of Orthopedics and Pediatrics
Department of Orthopedics
University of Texas Health Science
Center at San Antonio
7703 Floyd Curl Drive
US-78284-7774 San Antonio, Texas

Authors

Peter Illing, MD
Childrens Hospital "Park Schönfeld"
Department of Pediatric Surgery
Frankfurter Strasse 167
DE-34121 Kassel

Prof Pierre Lascombes, MD
Hôpital Brabois Enfants
Rue du Morvan
FR-54511 Vandoeuvre

Foreword

Kaye E Wilkins

"Children's fractures all do well with nonoperative treatment" was the emphasis in the past. The pioneer in the treatment of pediatric orthopedic fractures, Dr Walter Blount, was very opposed to surgical intervention [1]. In his classic textbook published in 1955, he stated "Operations on supracondylar fractures are frequently followed by restricted motion". He went on to say, "The use of internal fixation, because conservative management fails, **is the way of an impetuous surgeon**". This dogma established nonoperative techniques as the standard for treating fractures in children for many years. Certainly, in 1955 when his textbook was published, the surgical management of children's fractures usually required the use of extensive invasive techniques with large incisions.

As time has passed, there has been a dramatic change in the management of children's fractures. Surgical management has become more widely accepted and utilized. This has not been because the present generation of surgeons managing children's fractures has become more **impetuous**. The increase in the use of surgical techniques has become accepted because of three major factors:
1. Improvement in technology,
2. Children's fractures heal rapidly, thus long-term rigid fixation is unnecessary,
3. Financial and social pressures.

Technology. Newer technology items such as image intensifiers, cannulated screws, more flexible implants, and power drills have enabled fracture fixation to be performed with minimal tissue disturbance. Thus, the procedures have become markedly less invasive. Previously, surgical treatment meant large incisions with more tissue damage.

Rapid healing. Since the fracture healing processes are much more rapid in children, the development of the natural stabilization processes of fracture healing eliminates the need for long-term immobilization. Children have more rapid return of muscle function and reestablish motion more readily. Long-term rigid stabilization techniques are rarely needed.

Financial and social pressures. A classic example in the past was the management of treating fractures of the femoral shaft. These children were often managed as inpatients in traction for weeks which was both expensive and debilitating. Inpatient hospitalization is very costly. With both parents usually employed, hospitalization also put social pressures on the family. Psychologically, children do better when managed in their home environment. Techniques were thus developed to stabilize these fractures so that the children could be discharged after minimal hospitalization.

To meet the need to mobilize the children more rapidly, minimally invasive techniques were developed and refined. The first techniques utilized were external fixators. While effective in managing many long bone fractures, they were not well accepted by the patients. There were the major problems of scar formation and local infection at the pin sites.

Intramedullary stabilization techniques became popular at about the same time. In adults, rigid intramedullary fixation has become widely accepted. However, for many biological reasons, this type of stabilization is not appropriate in the skeletally immature. The early attempts at intramedullary stabilization utilizing Rush rods or Steinmann pins did not produce satisfactory results. By making the intramedullary devices more flexible, they became very useful in the pediatric age group. Thanks to the work of the pioneers in France, Switzerland, and Germany, the concept of Elastic Stable Intramedullary Nailing (ESIN) was developed. This technique of utilizing flexible intramedullary nails has revolutionized the management of long bone fractures in the skeletally immature. The European orthopedic community has gained considerable experience in this technique. Two major textbooks have been produced, one in French [2] and a second in

German [3]. Thus, the European community has had the luxury of having access to reference works on the basic principles plus the experience of the wide use of ESIN. Unfortunately, the English speaking orthopedic surgeons have been handicapped by not having a reference source in English. They have had to depend on journal articles and some short courses for their guidance on the use of ESIN.

This manual will go far to correct that deficiency. Becoming accomplished in utilizing the techniques of ESIN in the English speaking orthopedic community has in the past carried with it a significant learning curve. The completeness of this publication in putting together the basic principles, the description of the use of the specialized instruments and the step-by-step description of the specific techniques for each fracture type will greatly decrease this learning curve. I predict that this work will become an excellent resource for those English speaking surgeons treating fractures in their skeletally immature patients.

The primary authors of each of the chapters have shared with the reader their wide experience with the ESIN techniques in a clear and concise manner. As is consistent with AO Publishing, this manual is well organized and easy to follow. I am honored to have been asked to provide editorial direction and advice in the production of this valuable resource.

Finally, it must be remembered that the majority of fractures in children can still be treated by nonoperative methods. However, for those fractures that will have a better outcome when stabilized surgically, this manual will provide guidance as to the most appropriate methods of utilizing the ESIN technique.

Kaye E Wilkins, MD
San Antonio, Texas

[1] **Blount WP** (1955) *Fractures in Children.* 2nd ed. Baltimore: Williams & Wilkins.

[2] **Metaizeau JP** (1988) *Ostéosynthèse de l'enfant par embrochage centro-médullaire élastique stable.* Montepellier: Sauramps Médical.

[3] **Dietz HG** (1997) *Intramedulläre Osteosynthese im Wachstumsalter.* München Wien Baltimore: Urban & Schwarzenberg.

Introduction

Hans-Georg Dietz, Peter P Schmittenbecher, Theddy Slongo, Kaye E Wilkins

This manual is dedicated to operative fracture treatment in children and will introduce the reader to a special technique called Elastic Stable Intramedullary Nailing (ESIN), which is today the treatment of choice for the majority of shaft fractures in the growing child, especially in those situations where conservative treatment would not be indicated.

Most of the techniques generally applied in adults like interlocking nailing or plating are not ideally suited to the treatment of children due, for example, to the risk of physis injury, and overgrowth.

The authors have become familiar with this method over a period of twenty years and it is a great pleasure to present the philosophy of the method, outline the technique, and offer advice on how to manage special situations and complications.

ESIN is recommended primarily for shaft fractures and all the possible indications and techniques will be presented. However, some special indications for metaphyseal and joint fractures also exist and these will be explained in detail, too. The manual starts by stating the biomechanical principles of fracture treatment on which ESIN technique is based. It goes on to explain the development of the method, the required equipment, the indications, planning the procedure including all surgical considerations, postoperative care and results, furthermore, the pitfalls and pearls will be set out for additional clarity. The practical use of ESIN will be illustrated with reference to a large number of typical fractures with multiple case presentations for every segment of the upper and lower extremities. Finally, extended indications for ESIN in terms of special or rare cases and pathological fractures will also be included.

In the first part we give a complete overview of the ESIN technique as applied to the upper and lower extremities. In the second part we show extended indications for ESIN in rare cases and pathological fractures.

This manual is intended for all pediatric, trauma, and orthopedic surgeons dealing with the operative treatment of childrens fractures. The book provides a lot of "hands on" and "how to use" information. It is to be regarded as a "manual" in the true sense of the word: you take it, find your case or a similar one, and inform yourself about the steps of the operative procedure as they are recommended by an international group of experienced users who are able to draw not only on their own experience, but also on the experience of others and advanced training gained by participation at numerous national and international workshops and courses.

x

Acknowledgements

The idea for a new book and the desire to write it often arise quite spontaneously. In contrast, its realization in terms of processing and production requires a great deal of planning, hard work, and mutual understanding.

Therefore, it is of great importance to the editors that they extend their thanks to all those who have helped to achieve this "standard work" on ESIN treatment of fractures in childhood.

In the first instance, our thanks go to the AO Organization, especially AO Publishing, who offered us the opportunity to write this book in the first place.

For their active support and guidance, we would particularly like to thank Miriam Uhlmann, Project Coordinator for her untiring commitment to the project, Hanna Jufer, illustrator, for her masterly, child-specific drawings, and Urs Rüetschi, Head of AO Publishing.

We also wish to thank our two guest authors, Peter Illing and Pierre Lascombes, for their collaboration.

A book is only easy and pleasant to read if the phraseology is as perfect as possible and the text is correctly written and so a special and heartfelt thankyou goes to Kaye Wilkins and his wife for their dedicated and professional revision and editing of our texts. It is a particular honor for us to be able to include the name of Kaye Wilkins in our list of editors.

Hans-Georg Dietz, Peter Schmittenbecher, Theddy Slongo

Table of contents

1 Basic principles   **1**
2 Case collection of humeral fractures   **21**
3 Case collection of elbow fractures   **45**
4 Case collection of forearm fractures   **71**
5 Case collection of femoral fractures   **109**
6 Case collection of tibial fractures   **149**
7 Case collection of special indication fractures   **171**
　Appendix   **225**

1 Basic principles

1.1 Biomechanics 1
1 Basics of elastic stable intramedullary nailing (ESIN) in children 1
2 Biomechanical principles 2
3 Biomechanical properties 4
4 Special techniques designed to improve the biomechanics 7
5 Adaptation of the biomechanical principles to different approaches 9
6 Suggested reading 14

1.2 Implants and instruments 15
1 Implant designs and properties 15
2 Instruments 16

1.1 Biomechanics

1 Basics of elastic stable intramedullary nailing (ESIN) in children

1.1 What is ESIN?

Stability plus mobility
Elastic stable intramedullary nailing (ESIN) is a minimally invasive and minimally traumatic surgical technique designed to treat fractures in children. Stabilization is achieved with flexible intramedullary nails that have been precontoured to provide some elastic properties (Fig 1.1-1). This enables them to provide sufficient stability to permit early movement and partial weight bearing. Thus, ESIN is a biological and child-friendly method of osteosynthesis for transverse, oblique, and short spiral diaphyseal fractures in the immature skeleton.

Metaphyseal usage
The method is also suitable for the treatment of some special metaphyseal fractures such as:
- Radial neck fractures
- Proximal and distal metaphyseal-epiphyseal fractures of the humerus
- Proximal and distal metaphyseal fractures of the femur

1.2 Biology

Why is this technique biological and child friendly?

Rapid healing
The success of the ESIN technique is largely due to the fact that it produces less adverse effects on the healing of the fracture and the growth processes than other more invasive methods. Because of the elastic properties of the nails, this system supports the biology of children's fracture healing by stimulating both periosteal and endosteal callus formation (Fig 1.1-2).

Since this is a minimally invasive technique, the periosteum is respected and preserved. Cutting or stripping the periosteum, which usually occurs with any open procedure, has a deleterious effect on healing—it slows down both the speed of healing and callus formation. This slowing of the reparative processes, can in turn affect the length of the extremity by delaying the stimulation of growth associated with the healing process.

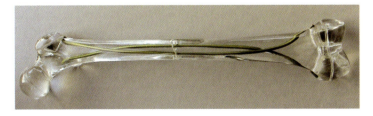

Fig 1.1-1 This model demonstrates the ideal positioning and curvature of the nails in the treatment of a midshaft fracture of the femur.

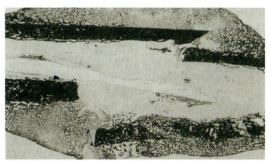

Fig 1.1-2 Histological view of periosteal and endosteal callus formation after ESIN. (Reproduced with kind permission of Métaizeau JP, Ostéosynthèse chez l'enfant; Sauramps Medical 1988.)

1 Basic principles

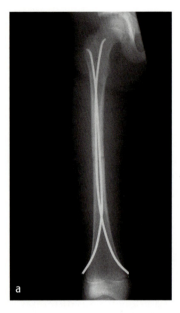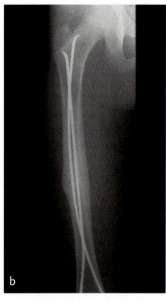

Fig 1.1-3a–b   AP and lateral x-rays at 4 months postoperative demonstrating almost complete remodeling of the callus.

Preserved periosteum
Since the fracture is usually managed in closed technique, ESIN produces a more normal biological environment by minimizing the periosteal damage. Even when an open reduction is required, the surgical incision over the fracture zone is minimal, being no more than is necessary to facilitate the reduction.

Micromotion
The elasticity of the two properly bent nails permits an ideal micromotion which enhances the rapidity of fracture healing (Fig 1.1-3).

The decrease in the healing time combined with the adequacy and stability of the fracture reduction helps to reduce the consolidation and remodeling time. This in turn decreases the temporal aspect of the healing process. This explains why less overgrowth has been observed in those patients treated with the ESIN techniques. Elastic nailing reduces and adequately stabilizes diaphyseal and metaphyseal fractures in terms of length, rotation, and alignment.

The reduction must be "anatomical" in as much as it corresponds to the respective remodeling capacity based upon the age of the child and the localization of the fracture.

To achieve a successful outcome, it is imperative that the treating surgeon acquires the basic knowledge to correctly apply this method.

2   Biomechanical principles

2.1   Basic properties

The elastic nails used to stabilize children's long-bone fractures, whether of titanium alloy or of stainless steel, have adequate strength to maintain the reduction until the fracture has healed. It should be noted that ESIN is a successful method for treating children's fractures because they heal rapidly in less than half the time of an equivalent adult fracture.

2.2   Precontour

It is recommended that the nails are precontoured in order to achieve 3-point contact. The degree of curvature of the nail should be approximately 3 times the diameter of the bone at the fracture site (Fig 1.1-4). Adding more of a curve with precontouring can increase the contact force on the inner cortex. This can be a definite advantage in the stabilization of unstable fractures.

1.1 Biomechanics

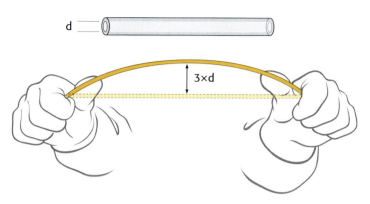

Fig 1.1-4 Precontouring the nails to 3 times the diameter of the diaphysis with maximal curvature at the level of the fracture.

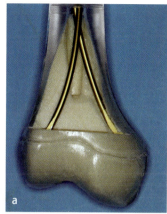 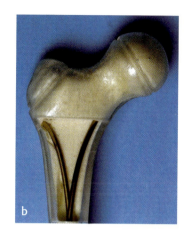

Fig 1.1-5a–b Good anchorage of both the tips of the nails in the metaphyses is essential to enhance stability.

Some authors do not precontour the nails before insertion, allowing the nails to become self-contoured during the process of insertion. However, experimental studies have demonstrated that a longer contact area of the nails with the inner cortex as well as a higher "spring effect" can increase the axial stability by a factor of 15 (see Tab 1.1-1). The apex of the curvature should be at the level of the fracture. Thus, when fractures are not in the midshaft, it may be easier to place the apex at the appropriate location by precontouring the nail.

2.3 Stability factors

In the vast majority of cases two nails of the same diameter are used. These need to be identically precontoured and inserted opposite each other in order to produce a perfectly balanced construct to maintain alignment. It is also imperative that there is good anchorage of both the tips and the ends of the nails in their respective proximal and distal metaphyses (Fig 1.1-5). Another feature that makes this method primarily suitable for children's fractures is the density of the bone in their metaphyses. Because of the stability provided by the nails in their respective metaphyses, they resist the tendency to be straightened. This, in turn, increases the tension within the intramedullary canal and, likewise, resists the tendency for further deformation.

2.4 Role of soft tissues

Part of the biomechanical stability of fractures stabilized by ESIN is provided by the intact muscle and other soft-tissue envelopes surrounding the affected bone. Thus, ESIN is particularly effective for closed fractures of the femur and forearm.

Multifragmentary fractures and fractures associated with extensive soft-tissue loss or stripping, such as Gustilo type III open tibial fractures, may be more difficult to stabilize with ESIN alone. In these situations, ESIN may need to be supplemented by a temporary external fixator or a splint.

1 Basic principles

2.5 Special conditions

Occasionally, three nails are introduced into a single long bone. It should be noted that this can upset the balance of the bipolar matched construct. Therefore, it should be used only to resist an excessive external deforming force such as a spastic muscle. There are conditions where it is advisable to use three nails, for example, in the proximal femur (see Fig 7.3-7, Fig 7.3-8, Fig 7.3-9 in chapter 7.3 Pathological femoral fractures). These are special situations where the basic biomechanical principles do not apply.

3 Biomechanical properties

The biomechanical principle of ESIN is based on the symmetrical bracing of two elastic nails inserted into the metaphysis, each supporting the inner cortical contact. This produces the following four biomechanical properties:
- Bending/bowing stability
- Axial stability
- Translational stability
- Rotational stability

All are essential to achieving an optimal result.

■■ The above properties only conditionally apply to the treatment of metaphyseal fractures. Only by adhering to the basic principles can sufficient support or stability be achieved in the metaphyseal areas. The surgeon should, however, apply these basic principles as much as the individual fracture pattern will allow.

The following two basic concepts must always be kept in mind:

1. Tension within the nail provides a "memory effect".
2. The elastic nails provide stability against external forces.

3.1 Stability factors

Axial stability
The rebound forces of the nails tend to bring the fragments back to the original position. To achieve this axial stability optimally, it is necessary that the nails have a long contact area with the inner cortex. The nails must form a kind of "parallelogram" along the fracture zone. When axial strain is applied, the inner pressure on the cortex will increase (Fig 1.1-6).

Translational stability
The parallel position of the nails also serves to resist translational displacement.

The longer the contact area of the nails at the inner cortex, the greater is the resistance to translational displacement (Fig 1.1-7, Tab 1.1-1). In turn, this enhances the optimal construction of the parallelogram.

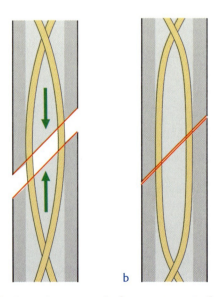

Fig 1.1-6a–b Long inner-cortical contact contributes to stability in the axial plane.

1.1 Biomechanics

Rotational stability

The elastic nails also achieve stability against rotational external forces (Fig 1.1-8). Even in unstable fractures, the nails must be well secured in the proximal and distal metaphyses.

3.2 Factors leading to failure

Failures of the surgeon

In general, it looks very simple to hammer two elastic nails into a bone. Because of the fact that fractures almost always heal in the child, the surgeon may have a tendency to omit some of the important aspects of the treatment necessary for success. Often the failure analysis of this method demonstrates the absence of adherence to the basic biomechanical principles. Unfortunately, in situations where this occurs it is usually the surgeon's mistake and not the fault of the method.

Most failures occur for the following reasons:
- Wrong indication as to the type or localization of the fracture or age and weight of the child
- Incorrect size of the nails: choosing the wrong diameter (ie, too thin) or using nails of different diameters
- Wrong technique: choosing different levels for the entry points or producing the so-called corkscrew phenomenon
- Failure by omission: not respecting the biomechanical principles of ESIN

These specific mistakes are demonstrated and discussed in detail in Fig 1.1-9.

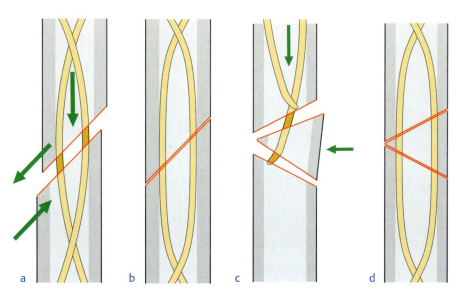

Fig 1.1-7a–d Translational stability. The parallel position of the nails provides resistance to translocation as well, even in multifragmentary fractures.

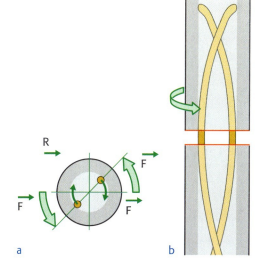

Fig 1.1-8a–b Rotational stability. Rotational rebound forces bring the fragments back into the correct position.

1 Basic principles

Failure to evaluate patterns
Individual failures may also occur if the pattern of the fracture is not taken into consideration. Specific examples include:
- Different levels of the entry points: This often produces different contact with the inner cortex leading to different strength of the nails which can result in axial deviation.
- Choosing nails of inadequate thickness: This can also contribute to a loss of the fracture stability producing malalignment (Fig 1.1-10) (too thin nails = loss of stability; too thick nails = loss of elasticity).
- Use of only one nail: This is not in keeping with the basic biomechanical principles and thus cannot be considered a stable system.

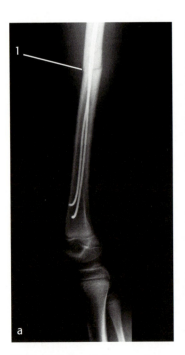
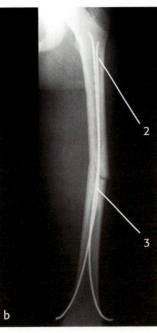
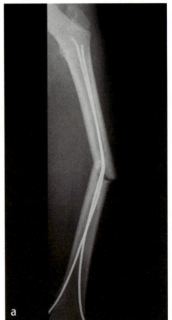
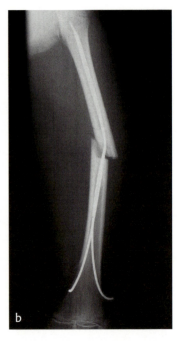

Fig 1.1-9a–b This case demonstrates a combination of different failures in the same patient. There is a failure of technique as manifested by a lack of cortical contact because of failure to precontour the nail (1). The nail diameters are too small (2). In addition there is a corkscrew phenomenon (3).

Fig 1.1-10a–b Loss of alignment. Because of failure to choose nails of adequate diameters, there is a loss of stability. This results in substantial deformation of the nails with weight bearing.

4 Special techniques designed to improve the biomechanics

4.1 Maintaining the advantages of ESIN

ESIN permits adequate stabilization of almost all diaphyseal fractures in patients aged 4–14 years. Nevertheless, certain well-known problems in the treatment of very long spiral fractures and multifragmentary fractures remain. By taking all biomechanical principles into account and adhering to the correct technique, these problems can largely be avoided.

4.2 Causes of instability

Insufficient stability may occur in the following circumstances:
- Older and tall children
- Physically disabled children with spastic or paralytic disorders
- Complex fractures in smaller children
- The fracture zone to be addressed is situated in the proximal or distal third
- Lack of anchorage in osteoporotic bones

4.3 Adaptations to increase the internal pressure

The question arises as to whether it is possible to improve the biomechanics of ESIN. Yet unpublished research carried out at the AO Research Institute in Davos, Switzerland, has shown that additional spreading at the intersection point of the nails can increase the inner pressure so much that the axial stability increases by a factor of 65 (Tab 1.1-1, Fig 1.1-11). The model used was the so-called "gap model" that simulated the situation of a completely unstable fracture.

Locking device	Axial compression (N)	Bending (Nm/deg)	Torsion 45°
No locking	10 N	0.18 Nm/deg	0 Nm
2–2.5 mm K-wires	350 N	0.22 Nm/deg	
2–2.5 mm threaded K-wires	350 N	0.18 Nm/deg	
2–3.5 mm screws	650 N	0.26 Nm/deg	0.38 Nm

Tab 1.1-1 Effects of increasing nail spread at crossing points.

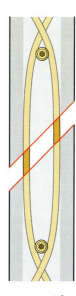

Fig 1.1-11 Test arrangement with 3.5 mm screws.

1 Basic principles

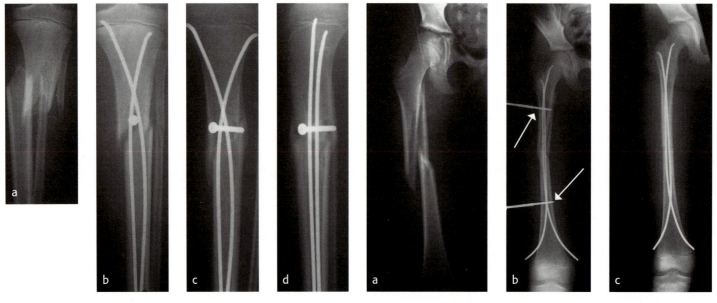

Fig 1.1-12a–d Miss-a-nail technique. Fracture of the proximal third of the tibia stabilized by ESIN. To increase the stability by changing the crossing point to a more proximal location, a 3.5 mm cortex screw was used in miss-a-nail technique.

Fig 1.1-13a–c External fixation supplementation. A patient with cerebral palsy and epilepsy sustained a long unstable spiral wedge fracture of the femur. The alignment was easily accomplished with two nails. To prevent shortening a small external fixator was applied to the screws placed in each of the apices on the diaphyseal side of the crossing points (arrows) for 3 weeks.

4.4 Increase internal pressure—miss-a-nail technique

Additional spreading to increase the pressure on the inner cortex can be achieved:
- Insertion of a 3.5 mm cortex screw close to either one or both of the proximal or distal apices on the diaphyseal side of the crossing point (Fig 1.1-12).
- Insertion of a 3.0 mm or 4.0 mm self-drilling, self-tapping Schanz screw into the apices on the diaphyseal side of the crossing points and connection via a small external fixator rod (Fig 1.1-13).

The holes for the screws should be drilled with Steinman pins and not a drill bit to lessen the chance of injuring the flexible nails.

1.1 Biomechanics

Cannulated screws should be used to facilitate later removal.

These are methods of simulating reinforced precontouring to increase the pressure against the inner cortices.

Thus, the length, rotation, and angulation can be optimally stabilized. The advantages lie in immediate, unproblematic mobilization and partial weight bearing. In physically handicapped patients, general care and positioning in the wheelchair is immediately possible.

Since adequate callus formation can be expected within 2–3 weeks of biological treatment with ESIN, the small external fixator, if applied, can be removed at this time. Stability is then completely assured.

If screws were inserted, they should be extracted first at the time of nail removal.

The miss-a-nail technique offers the option of expanding the indications for the ESIN method. It needs to be mentioned that this technique is used in a similar way with other products, such as special nails that have an eyelet at the end of the nail. However, these nails can be applied only in very special circumstances. Another option to increase stability is to use the end cap (see Fig 1.2-2).

5 Adaptation of the biomechanical principles to different approaches

To be able to appropriately treat all diaphyseal fractures, the surgeon must be able to adapt the standard techniques. However, if the technique is amended, it is always important to adhere to the basic biomechanical principles. Some of the fracture patterns have unique features. This requires learning which specific adaptations of the basic principles are essential for their treatment.

5.1 Single-side nail insertion

The most substantial adaption is required for those fractures where it is only possible for the nails to be inserted into the bone from one side (but through different insertion sizes). This is especially relevant to fractures of the distal and proximal humerus and distal femur.

S-shape configuration

When both nails are inserted on one side only, one of these nails must be rotated by 180° during the introduction process to produce the S-shape (Fig 1.1-14). This S-shape configuration is necessary when managing the humerus in both antegrade and retrograde insertion techniques combined with single-side insertion (Fig 1.1-15, Fig 1.1-16).

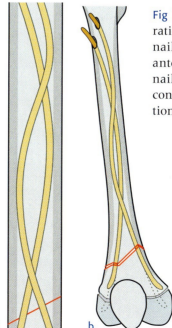

Fig 1.1-14a–b S-shape configuration. The first precountered nail is normally advanced in the antegrade direction. The second nail is changed into an S-shape configuration during its insertion process.

1 Basic principles

5.2 Wide separation of tips

In the very distal fractures in the metaphysis, it is important, that rigid stabilization of the tips is obtained. In other words, the tips need to be securely placed in good metaphyseal bone.

This is because the apex of the contoured portion does not lie within the fracture zone. Placing the tips in widely separated areas of rigid metaphyseal bone provides optimal stabilization for the fracture (Fig 1.1-15, Fig 1.1-16).

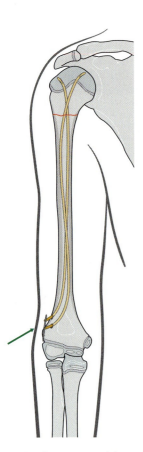

Fig 1.1-15   Correct position of the nails using the retrograde monolateral bracing at the humerus. Note the separation of the apices at the fracture site and the nail tips in the proximal metaphysis.

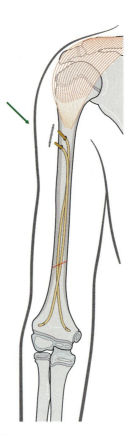

Fig 1.1-16   Correct position of the nails and bending apices using the antegrade monolateral bracing at the humerus. Again the bending apices are separated at the fracture site

1.1 Biomechanics

Obtaining an S-shape during manipulation

To obtain this special inner bracing, the first nail is inserted using the standard technique (Fig 1.1-17a). Through a second insertion site, the second nail, which has been appropriately prebent in the distal third, is inserted (Fig 1.1-17b). After this precontoured portion has been inserted completely into the medullary canal, the nail is rotated a full 180° (Fig 1.1-17c). It is important at this point to take care that the first nail is not crossed twice. The portion of the nail still remaining outside the bone is now bent forcefully in the longitudinal axis. This maneuver produces the desired S-shape. The use of this technique to produce the second curve of the S-shape (Fig 1.1-17d) during the manipulation process makes the insertion process easier than if this second curve was precountered.

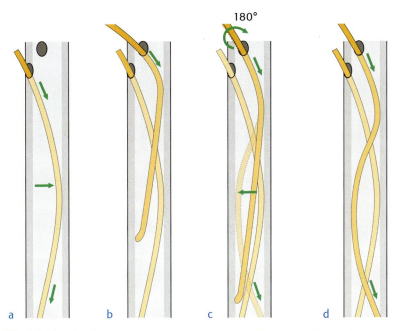

Fig 1.1-17a–d The step-by-step description of single-sided nail insertion and S-shape configuration.

Pitfalls −

As a rule, the good-naturedness of the method forgives many failures. However, errors may add up. For example, if you have an improper indication combined with the wrong technique, the result could be a major problem, such as a delayed union, a malunion, or severe shortening.

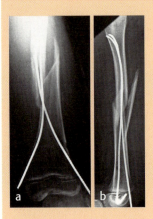

Fig 1.1-18a–b Different technical errors leading to failure are demonstrated in these AP and lateral x-rays:
- The approach is incorrect. The entry points are too high. The tips of the nails are in the wrong position.
- There is inadequate fixation because of a lack of 3-point contact. Distally, there is no nail contact. The crossing point is at the level of the fracture. There is a "corkscrew phenomenon" as manifested by three crossings of the nails.
- There is a lack of stability because the two nails have no contact with the inner cortex. These technical errors have led to failure as manifested by severe shortening.

Pearls +

It has been emphasized repeatedly that long spiral and completely unstable fractures cannot be treated sufficiently with ESIN. If however, all biomechanical principles are followed correctly and the techniques described above are applied, a proximal spiral fracture with spiral wedge can be treated adequately.

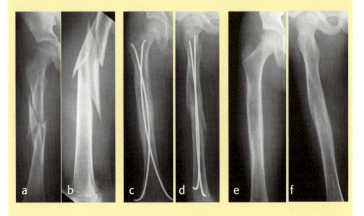

Fig 1.1-19a–f The fracture pattern in this femur involved the middle to proximal 1/3 with a spiral wedge (32-D/5.2). This is an absolutely unstable fracture. However, by strictly applying the basic principles of the ESIN technique, an excellent outcome has been achieved.
a–b Injury x-rays, AP and lateral views.
c–d AP and lateral views after 4 weeks show alignment with good callus bridging.
e–f Follow-up x-rays at 10 months after implant removal, demonstrating complete remodeling AP and lateral.

1.1 Biomechanics

Pitfalls − (cont)

Reduction and fixation
The most frequent pitfalls are:
- Shortening because of insufficient axial stability
- Rotational failures resulting from not comparing the postoperative rotation to that of the nonfractured extremity
- Leaving ends of the nails too long; this can produce skin perforation leading to a subsequent infection
- Axial deviation as a result of instability caused by
  – too thin nails,
  – corkscrew phenomenon,
  – the insertion points of the nails at different levels,
  – different sizes of the nails,
  – different nail curvatures

Rehabilitation
If there is inadequate stability, the child cannot be properly mobilized.

If shortening occurs, a second operation may be necessary. If the fracture is unstable, external stabilization in the form of a cast or splint may be needed.

Pearls + (cont)

Reduction and fixation
The following steps are essential:
- Good prebending of the nails, especially the tips
- The more proximal the fracture site, the greater is the need to precontour the nail in its distal third
- By doing this, the length of the inside contact can be extended. In addition, this shifts the crossing point to a more proximal position.
- The nails should not crisscross repeatedly (ie, producing a "corkscrew phenomenon")
- Miss-a-nail technique
- Additional small external fixator
- End caps

Rehabilitation
When the correct treatment is applied, no additional immobilization for either the lower extremity or the upper extremity is needed. Functional postoperative management is absolutely mandatory. The child should be able to return to his or her normal activities as soon as possible.

1 Basic principles

6 Suggested reading

Bräten M, Terjesen T, Rossvoll I (1993)
Torsional deformity after inramedullary nailing of femoral shaft fractures. Measurement of anteversion angles in 110 patients.
J Bone Joint Surg Br; 75(5):799–803.

Clinkscales CM, Peterson HA (1997)
Isolated closed diaphyseal fractures of the femur in children: comparison of effectiveness and cost of several treatment methods.
Orthopedics; 20(12):1131–1136.

Flyn JM, Hresko T, Reynolds RA, et al (2001)
Titanium elastic nails for pediatric femur fractures: a multi-center study of early results with analysis of complications.
J Pediatr Orthop; 21(1):4–8.

Linhart WE, Roposch A (1999)
Elastic stable intramedullary nailing for unstable femoral fractures in children: preliminary results of a new method.
J Trauma; 47(2):372–378.

Metaizeau JP (1988)
Ostéosynthèse chez l'enfant Embrochage centro-médullaire élastique stable. Montpellier, Saurarnps Médical.

Schmittenbecher PP, Dietz HG, Linhart WE, et al (2000)
Complications and Problems in Intramedullary Nailing of Children`s Fractures. *European Journal of Trauma;* 6:287–293.

Sola J, Schoenecker PL, Gordon JE (1999)
External fixation of femoral shaft fractures in children: enhanced stability with the use of an auxiliary pin.
J Pediatr Orthop; 19(5):587–591.

1.2 Implants and instruments

The ESIN method has three unique qualities:
1. It involves the use of a simple implant.
2. The technique is achieved with a simple method.
3. It requires only simple instruments.

1 Implant designs and properties

Dual function: implant/tool
The elastic nail plays a particular role. This special role of the nail lies in the fact that, in contrast to other methods, the nail is primarily a tool and only secondarily does it function as an implant. This is indeed a unique situation which is not seen in other systems of orthopedic instrumentation.

■ ■ **Preserving individual structure**
It is important that excessive manipulations during the introduction or advancement of the nail are avoided. Too much manipulation of the nail can completely alter its structure and biomechanical qualities. The same may occur with the indirect reduction of the fracture fragments. As a result, the stabilizing properties of the nails may be lost. Therefore, it is of great importance that the surgeon carefully follows the principles and techniques during the reduction and stabilization procedures.

Tip of the nail
The special bend of the tip of the nail allows it to glide more easily. The form of the tip also insures that the nail hits and glides well at an appropriate angle on the contralateral cortex.

The height of the tip of the nail is adjusted to match the diameter of the nail. This guarantees that the height of the tip will also fit properly within the medullary canal.

End of the nail
The tip of the nail corresponds with a marking at the end of the nail. Both are directed anteriorly on the nail. This orientation is provided so the direction of the tip can be determined without image intensification.

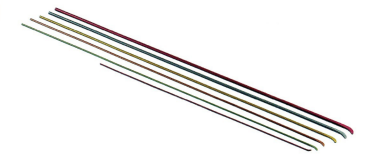

Fig 1.2-1   Nail sizes.
Nails are available in diameters of 1.5–5.0 mm. There are also nails with smaller diameters available. The heights of the individual nail tips vary and are determined by the diameter of the nail.

Length of the nail
Nails are available up to 45 cm. Nails of some producers have an unique length. Thus, preoperatively the desired length of the nails does not need to be determined. This allows for more precise placement of the nails. Other nailing systems are available with different standard nail lengths according to the nail diameter.

1 Basic principles

End caps (Fig 1.2-2)

With very unstable fractures in older children the axial stability can be improved by using end caps in critical situations. The use of end caps or similar mechanisms in situations with axial instability can help to prevent shortening. This is usually accomplished with a drill hole at the end of the nail for locking. To provide these alternative mechanisms the nails have to be of predetermined lengths

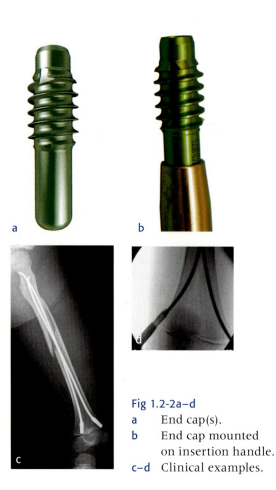

Fig 1.2-2a–d
a   End cap(s).
b   End cap mounted on insertion handle.
c–d   Clinical examples.

2 Instruments

Because of the uniqueness of the system, special instruments are recommended. To properly insert these implants, it is important that the necessary instruments are available in the operating room.

Handling and insertion of the implants can fundamentally be improved and simplified with the help of the instruments specifically designed for ESIN technique. Furthermore, the instruments have been carefully designed so as to reduce the time and amount of direct exposure required with the image intensifier.

The following are illustrated examples of the specialized instruments utilized to both insert and/or remove the ESIN implants.

Awl (Fig 1.2-3)

This is the usual and most common instrument to open the medullary canal. Because the metaphyseal bone is soft, it is important to rotate the awl by hand more than 90° to produce an adequate opening in the bone. In hard bone (eg, distal humerus) it can be tapped in with a hammer or a drill can be used alternatively.

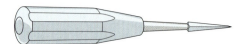

Fig 1.2-3   Awl for opening the bone.
The hand awl is used to create the insertion sites.

Inserter/T-handle (Fig 1.2-4)

The inserter is the primary instrument used with the nails. It facilitates nail guidance as it is inserted and advanced. It is constructed so that the hammer can strike directly on the flat surface of the handle.

⬛🟨 Hammer blows directly to the protruding inserter/T-handle must be avoided.

There are two special modifications in its construction that make nail insertion more smoother, thus decreasing image intensifier time.

1. The asymmetrical T-piece can be aligned with the tip of the nail to help with its orientation.
2. There are additional laser markings on the chuck to indicate the direction of rotation needed to tighten or loosen the chuck.

If this special inserter is not available, a normal T-handle chuck can be used.

Hammer (Fig 1.2-5)

The combined hammer (combination of a normal and a slotted hammer) can be used for insertion as well as for removal of the nails. The slotted part is normally used in combination with a hammer guide.

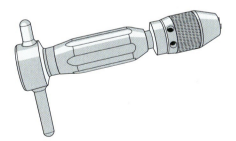

Fig 1.2-4   Inserter.
The hand chuck is used to hold the nails as they are inserted. The longer handle should be oriented in the same direction as the nail tip. The direction to open the chuck is laser printed on the chuck.

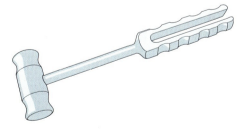

Fig 1.2-5   Hammer.
The combined hammer has a dual function. The head is used to advance the nails into the bone. The slotted shaft can be used with the hammer guide to extract the nails.

Hammer guide (Fig 1.2-6)

If a hammer is needed or the nail has to be moved forwards or backwards to reduce the fracture, a hammer guide is provided. This hammer guide can be screwed into the handle of the inserter. It is used as a guide for the slotted hammer (Fig 1.2-6b). Alternatively, the head of the hammer can be struck directly against the flat surface of the base of the hammer guide.

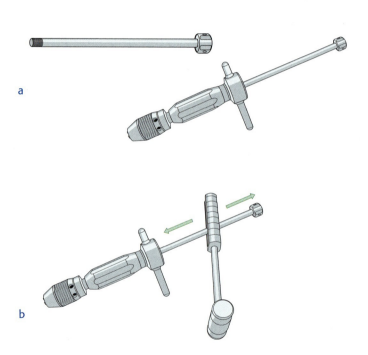

Fig 1.2-6a–b   Hammer guide.
It can be applied to the handle of either the chuck or extraction pliers.
a   The guide screws into the base of the handle.
b   The combination hammer can strike the guide base directly (arrow) to drive the nail into the bone. Alternatively, the hammer can be slid along the tube of the guide (arrow) to strike the top surface of the base for extraction of the nail.

Impactor (Fig 1.2-7)

A beveled impactor is provided for the definitive placement of the nail. The 8 mm hole and the beveled tip guarantees that the correct length of the nail protrudes from the cortex to ensure nail removal.

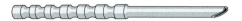

Fig 1.2-7   Impactor.
This device with a long tubular structure and a recessed hole in one end is used for the final impaction of the nail deep in the soft tissues when the hammer head can no longer be used. The flat end is used to drive in the nail over a long distance. The other end has an 8 mm hole and a beveled tip to ensure that the correct length of the nail protrudes from the cortex.

Nail cutter (Fig 1.2-8)

To shorten the nails a special cutting instrument is available. Care must be taken to ensure that the correct opening is used which corresponds to the proposed nail diameter. This nail cutter can be used very close to the skin without danger of damaging the soft tissues. If the special cutting instrument is not available, then a standard bolt cutter can be used. In this case the nail has to be cut outside the incision to prevent soft-tissue damage.

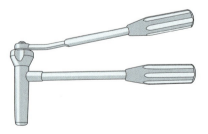

Fig 1.2-8   Nail cutter.
This device cuts the nails by a rotational motion of the handles. This allows the nail to be cut under or very close to the skin without injury to the wound margins.

Extraction pliers (Fig 1.2-9)

Removal of the nail can be very difficult. Therefore, it is important to have a good removal instrument. These special pliers are designed to be able to gain a good grip on the short protruding end of the nail. This is essential because of the forces required to extract a nail that was implanted for a long time. The handles of the pliers are constructed in such a way that the surgeon can use different methods to apply the extracting forces. The first option is to strike the hammer directly against the little protruding arm on the handle. The second option is to screw the hammer guide into the handle and use the slotted hammer. If these special extraction pliers are not available, ordinary flat-nosed pliers can be used.

F-tool (Fig 1.2-10)

This special tool can be used to indirectly apply reducing leverage forces to the surface of a limb suspended in traction to secure a final reduction. It is constructed of four radiolucent parts which form the letter F when put together. The main portion is a long thin rectangular piece with screw holes placed at strategic distances. There are three separate short round pieces that can be screwed into the holes depending on the thickness of the extremity. Two of these pieces are inserted into one end at the appropriate distance to lie on the anterior and posterior surfaces of the extremity. The other round piece is screwed into the other end protruding in the opposite direction. This piece can be used as a handle to apply the appropriate leverage force to the extremity and indirectly against the fracture ends to achieve the final reduction.

Alternative instruments

Alternatively, other instruments are available to apply the ESIN principles and techniques.

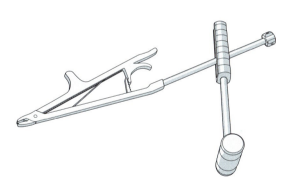

Fig 1.2-9   Extraction pliers.
This tool grasps the end of the nail very firmly to facilitate its extraction. The extracting force can be applied by either striking directly the protruding arm on the plier handle or using the slotted handle along the guide.

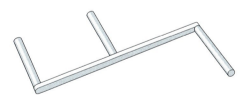

Fig 1.2-10   Radiolucent F-tool.
Leverage forces can be applied to the skin of the limb by raising the handle of this radiolucent tool. This brings the fracture fragments into a better alignment to facilitate nail passage.

2 Humerus

2.1 Introduction—humeral fractures 21
1. Indication 21
2. Patient preparation and positioning 21
3. Surgical principle 23
4. Implant removal 24
5. Suggested reading 24

2.2 Proximal humeral fracture, completely displaced (11-M/4.1) 25

2.3 Humeral shaft fracture, spiral, displaced, and unstable (12-D/5.1) 31

2.4 Humeral shaft fracture, transverse, displaced (12-D/4.1) 37

2.1 Introduction—humeral fractures

1 Indication

Subcapital humeral fractures
Age is not a factor in determining the indication for surgical stabilization of completely displaced fractures. In patients under 10 years, fractures with an axial deviation of more than 30° varus, ante- or recurvature, or more than 10° valgus need surgical stabilization to achieve and maintain adequate alignment.

In patients older than 10 years, any axial deviation of greater than 10° in any of the varus, ante- or recurvature planes is an indication for surgical stabilization. Other very specific indications would be in the management of pathological fractures (ie, juvenile bone cysts) or in the polytraumatized child to facilitate management in an intensive care unit setting (ICU).

Humeral shaft fractures
Fortunately, in the upper arm, malalignment rarely creates any functional loss. The flexibility of the shoulder allows most angular or rotational malalignment to be compensated.

However, because axial deviations of more than 10° tend to produce a cosmetically malaligned arm, surgical stabilization is often indicated. Other indications are:
- Fractures in polytraumatized children.
- Ipsilateral fractures of the humerus and forearm.
- Accompanying fractures of a lower extremity where there is need to use crutches.
- Open fractures Gustilo type II and III.
- Pathological fractures or any generalized disease that renders conservative treatment impossible.

Radial nerve dysfunction
The patient with a primary weakness of the radial nerve may benefit from surgical stabilization to facilitate the initiation of immediate physical therapy. However, an immediate open reduction of the fracture with nerve exploration is not indicated in this situation because there is usually spontaneous recovery of radial nerve function.

2 Patient preparation and positioning

Emergency treatment of these fractures is usually reserved for open fractures, vascular injuries, or general conditions where an immediate operation would be necessary.

Medication
Antibiotic prophylaxis is recommended for open fractures only. For closed fractures it should conform to the standard of care of clinical protocol.

Indications for thrombosis prophylaxis are limited to overweight children or postmenarchal girls taking birth control medication. Another indication would be if immobilization were necessary for general conditions such as polytrauma, injuries of the lower extremity or pelvis, or severe nontraumatic illness.

2 Humerus

2 Patient preparation and positioning (cont)

Patient positioning
The patient is placed supine with the injured extremity on an arm table (Fig 2.1-1a). In subcapital fractures the shoulder needs to be positioned inside the table to prevent the metal edge of the table interfering with the image. In shaft fractures the patient needs to be placed as lateral as possible so that an undisturbed image of the fracture region can be obtained.

Alternatively, the arm is positioned on the surgical table parallel to the patient's body (Fig 2.1-1b). This facilitates the entire process of image intensification which can be performed within the confines of the table for both subcapital and shaft fractures.

The entire upper extremity including the shoulder is prepared and draped. The hand is covered with a surgical glove. It is insufficient to prepare and drape out only the surgical entrance area around the elbow.

Equipment
- Standard ESIN set.
- Power drill.
  The use of a drill is optional, it might be necessary because perforation of the dense cortical bone of the distal humerus with an awl alone may be difficult to accomplish.
- Nails:
  – 2.0–3.0 mm stainless steel or titanium;
  – 1/3 of the diameter of the medullary canal at the mid-diaphyseal region.
  – Both nails must be of the same size.
  – Stainless steel nails are preferred in older children because the resistance to friction within the medullary canal of the humerus is very high.
- Image intensifier.

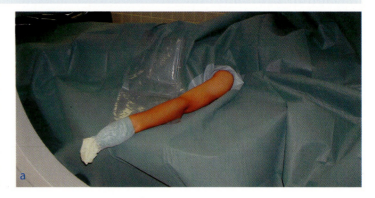

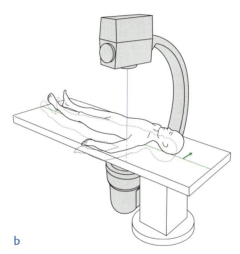

Fig 2.1-1a–b
a Positioning with an arm table. For shaft fractures the arm lies on the arm table.
b Positioning with the operating table. For subcapital fractures the shoulder should lie inside the table. All the imaging is performed inside the operating table.

2.1 Introduction—humeral fractures

3 Surgical principle

Direction of nailing in proximal fractures
Employ retrograde nailing using a lateral entry point distally as this requires only one incision with two entry points in the cortex (Fig 2.1-2a).

Direction of nailing in shaft fractures
In those fractures involving the middle and proximal third of the diaphysis, use retrograde nailing, employing both lateral and medial entry points (Fig 2.1-2b). In those involving the distal third of the diaphysis, use antegrade nailing through one single lateral subdeltoid approach for both nails with two entrance points in the cortex (Fig 2.1-2c).

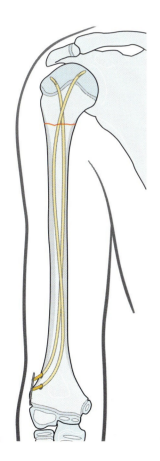
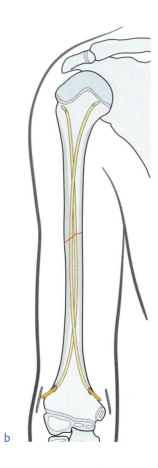
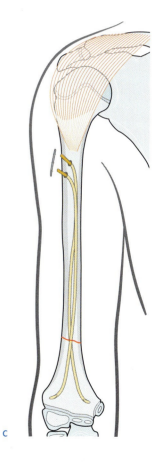

Fig 2.1-2a–c Nail insertion techniques.
a Retrograde one side (lateral).
b Retrograde both sides (medial and lateral).
c Antegrade one side (lateral).

4 Implant removal

Proximal fractures

If there was perforation of the epiphyseal plate, an x-ray is taken 6–8 weeks after surgery. If there is good bony consolidation, the nails can be removed (Fig 2.1-3).

Shaft fractures

X-rays are taken 3 months after surgery. If there is full consolidation and remodeling of the bone, the nails may be removed (Fig 2.1-4). If consolidation and remodeling are inadequate, then nail removal should be postponed. Premature removal should be performed only if there are skin irritation problems around the entrance points.

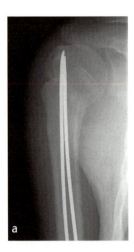 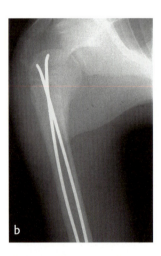 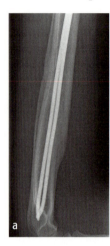 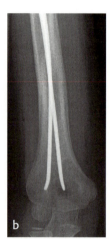

Fig 2.1-3a–b   X-ray of a subcapital fracture showing consolidation and remodeling.

Fig 2.1-4a–b   Lateral and AP x-rays of a shaft fracture showing consolidation and remodeling.

5 Suggested reading

Gautier E, Slongo T, Jakob RP (1992)
Treatment of subcapital humerus fracture with the Prevot nail.
Z Unfallchir Versicherungsmed; 85(3):145–155.

Havranek P, Pesl T (2002)
Use of the elastic stable intramedullary nailing technique in non-typical pediatric fractures.
Acta Chir Orthop Traumatol Cech; 69(2):73–78.

Machan FG, Vinz H (1993)
Humeral shaft fracture in childhood.
Unfallchirurgie; 19(3):166–174.

Schittko A (2003)
Humerus shaft fractures.
Unfallchirurg; 106(2):145–160.

Schmittenbecher PP, Blum J, David S, et al (2004)
Treatment of humeral shaft and subcapital fractures in children. Consensus report of the child trauma section of the DGU.
Unfallchirurg; 107(1):8–14.

Schwendenwein E, Hajdu S, Gaebler C, et al (2004)
Displaced fractures of the proximal humerus in children require open/closed reduction and internal fixation.
Eur J Pediatr Surg; 14(1):51–55.

Sessa S, Lascombes P, Prevot J, et al (1990)
Centro-medullary nailing in fractures of the upper end of the humerus in children and adolescents.
Chir Pediatr; 31(1):43–46.

2.2 Proximal humeral fracture, completely displaced (11-M/4.1)

1 Case description

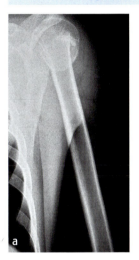
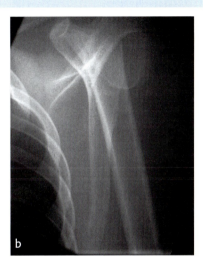

A 14-year-old male fell from a tree landing directly on his left shoulder. Clinically, he presented with significant swelling of the shoulder combined with painful restriction of motion. The x-rays demonstrated a closed completely displaced transverse fracture of the proximal metaphysis of the left humerus.

Fig 2.2-1a–b AP and transscapular Y x-rays of the fractured humerus.

2 Surgical approach

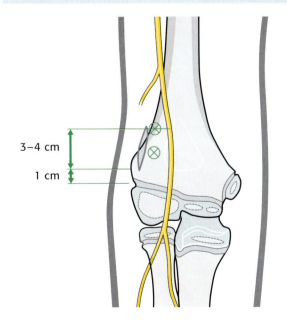

Skin incision
Incise the skin at the lateral aspect of the distal humerus. If possible, it is recommended that a medial entrance site should be avoided because of the risk of ulnar nerve injury. Begin the incision 1 cm above the palpable prominence of the lateral epicondyle and progress 3–4 cm proximally (cranially) up the lateral aspect of the humerus.

Approach
Spread the subcutaneous tissue to expose the fascia. Blunt dissection the fascia to expose the lateral supracondylar ridge of the distal humerus, taking care to remain on the anterior side of the intramuscular septum. Sharp opening of the periosteum and subperiosteal preparation to avoid injuring the radial nerve.

Fig 2.2-2 The skin is incised for 3–4 cm over the lateral aspect of the distal humerus starting about 1 cm proximal to the prominence of the lateral condyle.

2 Humerus

2 Surgical approach (cont)

Nail insertion

Once the bone is exposed, place an awl at the cranial end of the incision 90° to the lateral cortical surface. Care must be taken when drilling with the awl to avoid slipping off the lateral cortex. If the awl progresses easily into the lateral cortex, it is shifted cranially to a position of 45°. Progressively drill with the awl until it enters the medullary cavity (Fig 2.2-3).

Introduce the first nail and advance it proximally to the diaphyseal region. Drill with the awl a second time 1–2 cm caudal (distal) and approximately 1 cm anterior of the first insertion site. Lean the awl against the first nail to serve as a guide and keep it from slipping. Continue by drilling a second insertion site with the awl in the same manner as the first (Fig 2.2-4a).

Once this entrance site is completed, introduce the nail and advance it proximally to the diaphyseal region. If the cortical bone is very hard, a drill should be used to make the insertion sites.

Both nails are advanced proximally to lie just distal to the fracture site. It is very important to guide the nails so that they are not twisted one around the other (corkscrew phenomenon). The tips of the nails are directed at 90° to the fracture line (Fig 2.2-4b).

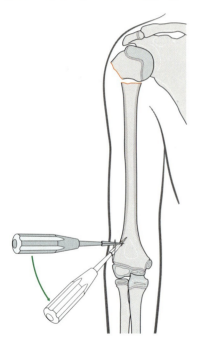

Fig 2.2-3   First entrance site.
This is usually the proximal site. The awl is started first at 90° until it engages the cortex. It is then gradually tilted to 45° as it drills through the cortex.

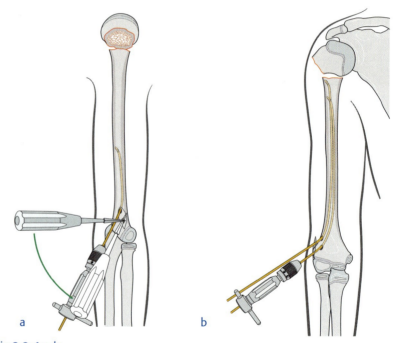

Fig 2.2-4a–b
a   First and second nail. The first nail is inserted through its entrance site and advanced proximally. The second entrance site is then made distally and anteriorly with the awl. The handle of the awl is leaned against the first nail to guide it until it has penetrated the cortex.
b   The second nail is inserted and both nails are advanced proximally to the fracture site.

2.2 Proximal humeral fracture, completely displaced (11-M/4.1)

3 Reduction and fixation

Reduction

Reduce the fracture by applying distal traction to the extended upper extremity. Using countertraction with a towel placed under the axilla, distal traction is continued until length has been reestablished. Fracture reduction is completed by abducting the arm to line up the fracture surfaces of the proximal and distal fragments (Fig 2.2-5a).

Stabilization

Once a satisfactory reduction has been achieved, advance the first nail proximally into the epiphysis without any concern about perforating the physis. Do not forget that on the AP image the humeral head is in an oblique position in relation to the shaft. If the position of the humeral head is not perfect, turn the nail to correct the position of the proximal fragment indirectly (Fig 2.2-5b). Sometimes it might be helpful to insert a nail percutaneously into the epiphysis and use it as a joystick to manipulate the epiphysis into the proper position.

Final placement

Make sure that the tips of the nails are in divergent positions. The positions of both nails are confirmed and nail perforation is excluded by taking the proximal humerus through a full range of motion using real time imaging. There needs to be free articular movement without any restriction. If the reduction and stability are satisfactory, the nails are cut distally so the tips lie deep within the subcutaneous tissue (Fig 2.2-5c).

The wound is closed with single sutures.

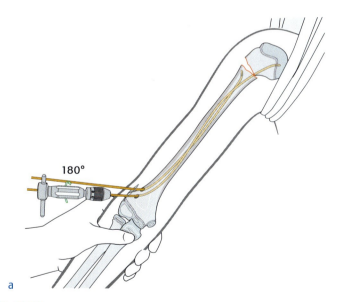
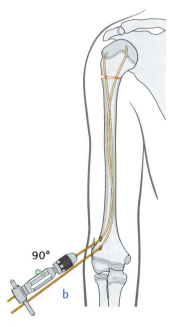
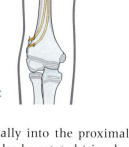

Fig 2.2-5a–c
a Reduction and fixation. The fracture is reduced by bringing the distal fragment into abduction. One nail is advanced into the proximal fragment. Some correction of the reduction can be achieved by rotating the second nail (circular arrow).
b The first nail is advanced proximally into the proximal fragment. The tip of this nail can also be rotated (circular arrow) to improve the fracture alignment.
c Final position. Once both nail tips have been secured in the head, the pins are cut distally. Notice the tips have the desired divergence.

4 Postoperative care and rehabilitation

Early motion

No additional external protection is necessary. Free movement is allowed immediately depending on the degree of postoperative pain with no restrictions concerning the range of motion.

The patient can be discharged after the x-rays have been taken on the first postoperative day to ensure that the reduction has been maintained (Fig 2.2-6a–b). No physiotherapy is required.

Healing

The first follow-up x-rays are taken at 4 weeks (Fig 2.2-6c–d). If there is adequate callus formation, then sports activities can be resumed. The final x-rays are taken 8 weeks later to check for full remodeling (Fig 2.2-6e–f). At this time implant removal can be planed as an outpatient procedure.

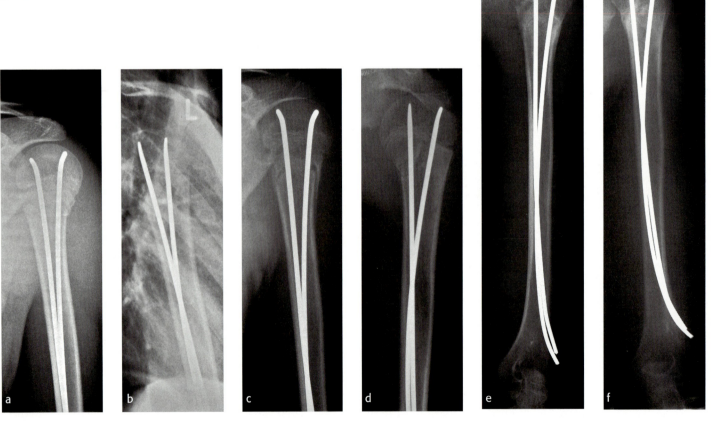

Fig 2.2-6a–f
- a–b Postoperative AP and lateral x-rays demonstrating excellent positioning of the nail tips in the proximal fragment.
- c–d AP and lateral x-rays at 4 weeks show early callus formation.
- e–f AP and lateral x-rays 8 weeks postoperatively demonstrate the matured callus.

2.2 Proximal humeral fracture, completely displaced (11-M/4.1)

4 Postoperative care and rehabilitation (cont)

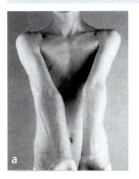
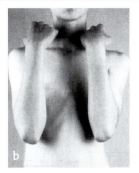
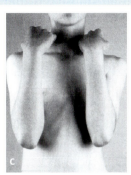

Fig 2.2-7a–c Motion reestablished. Three views taken at 12 weeks demonstrating full recovery of shoulder motion. Full physical activity is allowed.

5 Alternative case—type 12-D/4.1

Even in smaller children, exactly the same technique of intramedullary stabilization is useful. A 9-year-old boy fell from a tree sustaining an injury to his left shoulder area. X-ray taken in the emergency room revealed a completely displaced fracture at the proximal humeral diaphysis (Fig 2.2-8a).

The fracture was stabilized using the retrograde ESIN technique (Fig 2.2-8b). As the fracture healed, he was able to gain early recovery of both motion and strength in the upper extremity Fig 2.2-8c).

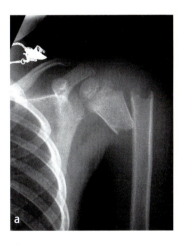
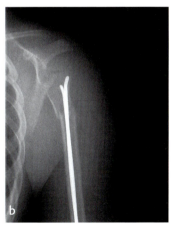
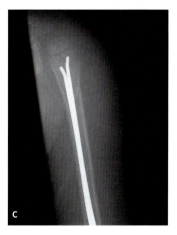

Fig 2.2-8a–c
a Displaced fracture of the proximal humeral diaphysis with shortening and bayonet apposition.
b Postoperative x-ray showing good reduction and placement of the nail tips.
c 8 weeks postoperatively sufficient callus is visible and nail removal can be considered.

6 Pitfalls –

Approach
Incision too proximal with the risk of radial nerve injury.

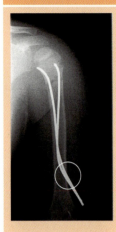

Fig 2.2-9 The high entry point of the nails resulted in a paresis of the radial nerve postoperatively and additionally one nail is perforating the cortex.

Reduction and fixation

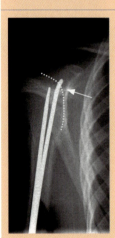

Fig 2.2-10 X-rays demonstrate a poor fit of the nail tips with penetration of the head (arrow and dotted line).

Rehabilitation
Fig 2.2-11 Nail ends are too long producing a risk of skin perforation and/or irritation with blockage of elbow flexion.

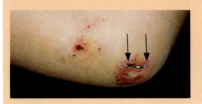

7 Pearls +

Approach
Fig 2.2-12 Especially in small children, start the skin incision 1 cm above the lateral epicondylar prominence to be as distal as possible from the radial nerve.

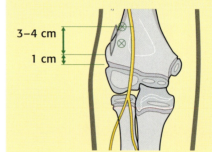

Reduction and fixation
Fig 2.2-13a–b Make sure the entire humeral head is inspected with the image intensifier. Rotate the upper extremity 180° to confirm that shoulder motion is free and complete.

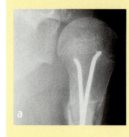 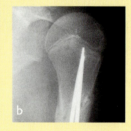

Rehabilitation
Sufficient cutting of the nails: it is best to withdraw the nails a few millimeters before cutting them and then reinserting them proximally.

2.3 Humeral shaft fracture, spiral, displaced, and unstable (12-D/5.1)

1 Case description

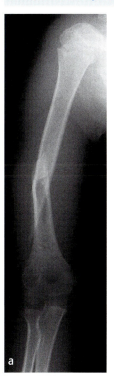
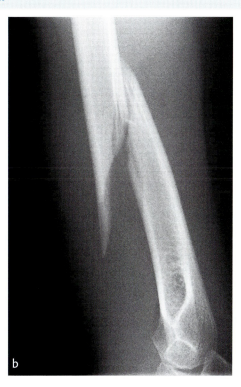

A 6-year-old girl fell breaking her fall with her right outstretched arm. The extremity was painful with an obvious displacement in the region of the humeral shaft. Clinically, there was intact skin with a functioning radial nerve.

X-rays demonstrated a spiral fracture extending from the middle to the distal third of the left humeral diaphysis. The fragments were displaced into antecurvature and varus (Fig 2.3-1). Clinically, this fracture pattern was felt to be unstable.

Fig 2.3-1a–b AP and lateral x-rays of the right arm showing a long spiral fracture of the humeral shaft with anterolateral apical angulation.

2 Surgical approach

Skin incision
Make a lateral 3–4 cm long incision at the caudal edge of the distal portion of the deltoid muscle. It is important not to incise too distally to avoid injuring the radial nerve. The subcutaneous tissue and the fascia are split to expose the bone.

Proximal insertion sites
Place the awl at the caudal end of the incision perpendicular to the bone to initiate drilling the first entrance hole. Once the awl engages the cortical bone, move it to a 45° angle to the long axis of the bone to enter the medullary canal (Fig 2.3-2a). Because the cortical bone in this area may be too hard to hand drill with the awl, an electric drill can be used to create the entrance sites.

Nail insertion
Introduce the nail into the medullary canal and advance it distally to the fracture region. Place the awl a second time against the bone 1–2 cm proximally and either a little anteriorly or posteriorly to the first perforation. Lean the awl against the first nail to guide it in the proper direction. Continue drilling the second entrance site with the awl to produce an oblique distally directed drill hole into the medullary canal. Insert the second nail (Fig 2.3-2b) and advance it distally to the fracture line. Rotate this second nail 180° so that the tip is directed medially and divergent to the first nail tip (Fig 2.3-2c).

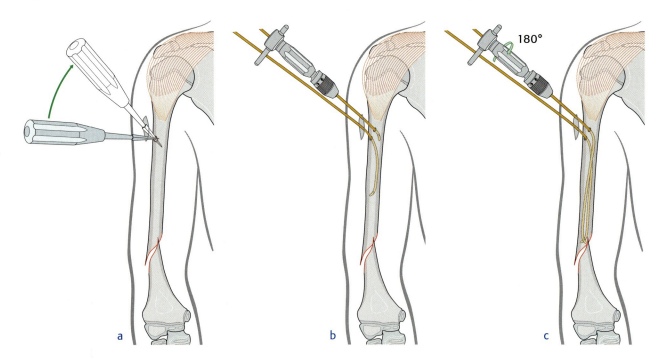

Fig. 2.3-2a–c   Primary nail insertion.
a   The incision is placed at the caudal distal edge of the deltoid muscle. An awl is used to create the entrance sites on the lateral and anterior surfaces of the cortex.
b   The nails are inserted into their respective entrance sites and advanced distally towards the fracture.
c   Once the fracture has been reached, the proximal nail is rotated 180° (circular arrow) so that its tip is divergent to that of the distal nail.

2.3 Humeral shaft fracture, spiral, displaced, and unstable (12-D/5.1)

3 Reduction and fixation

Direct and indirect reduction

The distal fragment is secured by the hand of an assistant who applies slight traction. Then the nails are used like handles to bring the proximal fracture surface into contact with that of the distal fragment by direct manipulation. While the reduction is being maintained, advance the more easily inserted nail into the distal fragment (Fig 2.3-3a). Attempt to improve the reduction by rotating the tip of the first nail to achieve an indirect reduction. Advance the second nail into the distal medullary canal (Fig 2.3-3b). To prevent any secondary radial nerve injury, take care that the nails do not leave the medullary canal through the fracture into the surrounding tissue.

Fracture stabilization

Now orient both nails correctly to prevent the corkscrew phenomenon and advance them distally to the radial and ulnar supracondylar columns (Fig 2.3-3c). Rotate the nails slightly to carefully align the exact positions of the apices of the tension bends so the alignment achieves a perfect spreading of the nails at the fracture level. Now secure the nails in the strong metaphyseal bone by a few hammer blows to the beveled impactor or directly on the nails ends. Finally, cut the nails and place the ends in the subcutaneous tissue. Close the skin with 1 or 2 single sutures (Fig. 2.3-3d).

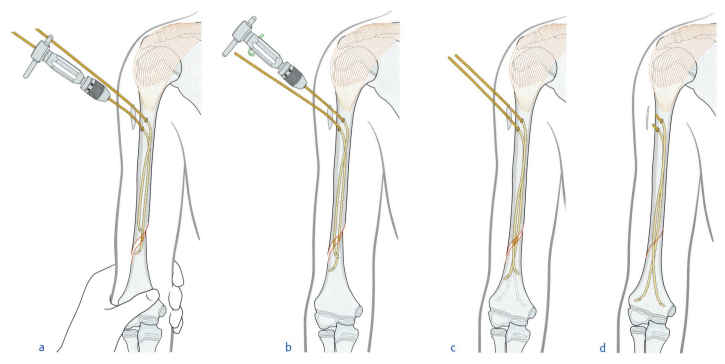

Fig. 2.3-3a–d   Reduction and stabilization.
a   As an assistant stabilizes the distal fragment, the nails are inserted into the proximal fragment. These nails can be used to manipulate this fragment to achieve a satisfactory reduction. Once reduced, one of the nails is advanced into the distal fragment.
b   The second nail is advanced across the fracture site.
c   The tips of both nails are advanced into the supracondylar columns. Final stabilization is achieved by driving the nail tips into the solid metaphyseal bone.
d   After the nails have been cut, the incision is closed with a few sutures.

2 Humerus

4 Postoperative care and rehabilitation

Because of the stability achieved, the child can begin unrestricted active shoulder motion immediately following surgery. No postoperative external support is needed. Normal postoperative pain and swelling causes some of the children to be reluctant to initiate much in the way of active motion for a few days. Prior to discharge postoperative x-ray documentation is accomplished (Fig 2.3-4a–b). Follow-up x-rays 4 weeks postoperatively should demonstrate sufficient callus to permit participation in sports activities (Fig 2.3-4c–d). 3 months after surgery, the callus should have undergone sufficient remodeling and be consolidated enough to consider nail removal (Fig 2.3-4e–f).

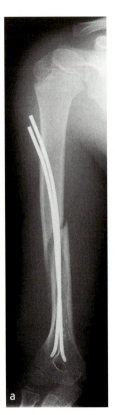
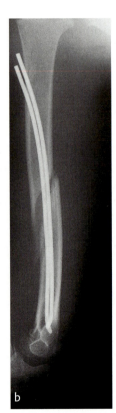
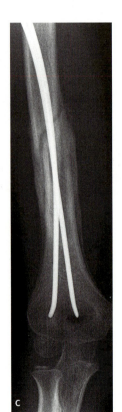
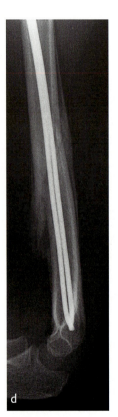
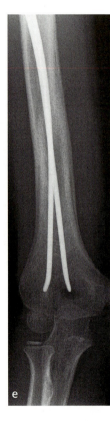
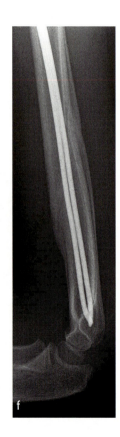

Fig 2.3-4a–f
- a–b AP and lateral x-rays at discharge demonstrate satisfactory positioning of the nails.
- c–d AP and lateral x-rays at 4 weeks postoperatively demonstrate good callus surrounding the fracture site.
- e–f X-rays taken 3 months postoperatively demonstrate sufficient healing and remodeling to consider nail removal.

2.3 Humeral shaft fracture, spiral, displaced, and unstable (12-D/5.1)

5 Pitfalls –

Approach
The subdeltoid entrance site in small children may be too close to the fracture site to permit stable reduction of the fracture.

Reduction and fixation
Insufficient spreading of the nails may inadequately align the fragments.

Iatrogenic radial nerve injury can result from:
- Injury by the nail(s) during insertion
- Fixation of the nerve within the fracture site

6 Pearls +

Approach
In small children sometimes it may be best to use a transdeltoid approach or an retrograde approach.

Reduction and fixation
At the end of the operation it is imperative to check the final position of the fragments with the image intensifier by real-time visualization. A final correction may be achieved by slight rotation of the nails.

If following the nailing procedure, there is postoperative radial nerve paralysis, the nail should be replaced. At the same time there should also be an open surgical inspection of the nerve.

| 5 Pitfalls – (cont) | 6 Pearls + (cont) |

Reduction and fixation (cont)
Spiral fractures of the humerus also can be stabilized faultlessly at a correct application of the ESIN technique.

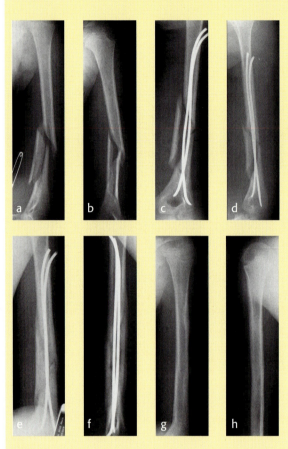

Fig 2.3-5a–h   13-year-old female with wring injury and nervus radialis irritation.
a–b   AP and lateral injury x-rays.
c–d   Postoperative x-rays.
e–f   Postoperative x-rays after 10 weeks.
g–h   Follow-up x-rays after 6 months.

2.4 Humeral shaft fracture, transverse, displaced (12-D/4.1)

1 Case description

A 13-year-old male was struck by a motor vehicle while riding his bicycle. He sustained a transverse midshaft fracture of the humerus. The fracture was unstable and displaced, producing a visible axial deformity of the arm.

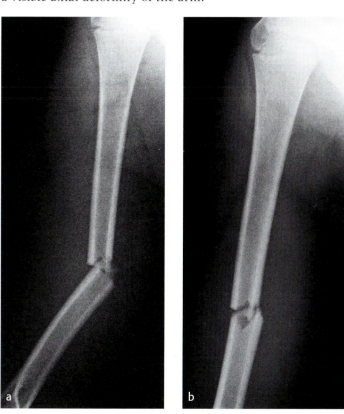

Fig 2.4-1a–b Preoperative AP and lateral x-rays showing an transverse, completely displaced humeral shaft fracture.

2 Surgical approach

Skin incisions
Symmetrical medial and lateral skin incisions are created starting 1 cm above the epicondylar regions and extending approximately 3 cm proximally.

Approach
After spreading the subcutaneous tissue and the fascia, place the awl at 90° to the bone at the upper edge of the incisions. Care must be taken to place the awl exactly on the lateral and medial edges of the bone. On the ulnar side, one must be aware that the distance from the skin surface to the bone is greater because of the accentuated ulnar waist of the humerus. Take care not to injure the ulnar nerve. On the radial side, it is important to always work distally in order to avoid injuring the radial nerve (Fig 2.4-2).

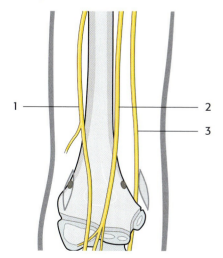

Fig 2.4-2 Anatomical location of the nerves. It is important to remember that three nerves run through this area:
1 Anterolateral—the radial nerve
2 Anteromedial—the median nerve
3 Posteromedial—the ulnar nerve

2 Humerus

2 Surgical approach (cont)

Entrance sites and nail insertion
Drill the cortical entrance sites, being careful that they are symmetrically placed. To enter the medullary canal, the awl is progressively brought to an oblique angle of 45° (Fig 2.4-3a).

Because of the sharpness of the edges of the humeral cortices in this area, one has to carefully control the awl so that it will not migrate either anterior or posterior. Introduce both nails and advance them proximally to the fracture line (Fig 2.4-3b–c).

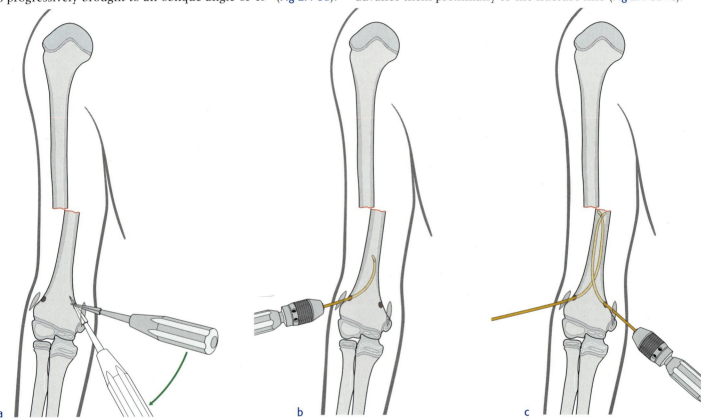

Fig 2.4-3a–c
a   The awl is used to carefully produce the entrance sites which should be symmetrically placed. Once seated in the cortical bone, the awl is then moved in a 45° angle, directed to enter the medullary canal of the distal humerus.
b   The lateral nail is inserted and advanced proximally in the medullary canal.
c   The second nail is then inserted and both nails are advanced proximally to the fracture.

2.4 Humeral shaft fracture, transverse, displaced (12-D/4.1)

3 Reduction and fixation

Direct and indirect reduction

The fracture is reduced by having the proximal fragment stabilized by an assistant and manipulating the distal fragment, using both nails like handles. After the fragment fracture surfaces have been brought into contact, the tip of one of the nails is advanced a few centimeters into the medullary canal of the proximal fragment (Fig 2.4-4a). An indirect reduction is performed by rotating this nail to bring the fracture surfaces into better apposition.

Nail placement

The second nail is then advanced into the proximal fragment (Fig 2.4-4b). Both nails are advanced up to the proximal metaphyseal area. It is important to ensure that the nails are not twisted around one another to avoid creating a corkscrew phenomenon. The correct alignment of both nails is achieved by slightly rotating them to place their bending apices directly opposite each other at the level of the fracture site. The nail ends are cut and buried in the subcutaneous tissue. The wounds are closed with one or two sutures (Fig 2.4-4c).

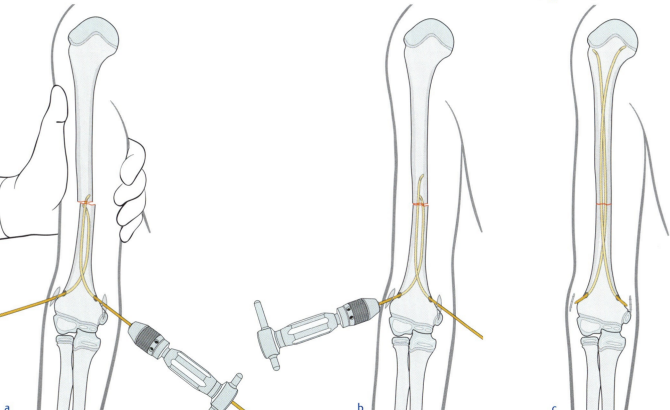

Fig 2.4-4a–c
- a The fracture is partially reduced by manual manipulation followed by advancement of the first nail into the proximal fragment.
- b The indirect reduction is completed by slightly rotating the nail and advancing the second nail.
- c Final position of the cut nails in which their bending apices are placed directly opposite each other at the fracture site.

4 Postoperative care and rehabilitation

Active motion of the extremity can begin immediately. On the following day just prior to discharge, x-rays are taken to confirm maintenance of the reduction (Fig 2.4-5a–b). At 4 weeks post injury, if there is sufficient callus formation on the x-rays, all activities including sports are allowed. Removal of the nails can be performed 3 months later if adequate consolidation and remodeling are demonstrated on the x-rays (Fig 2.4-5c–d). The guidelines for nail removal in pathological fractures can be found in chapter 7 Special indications.

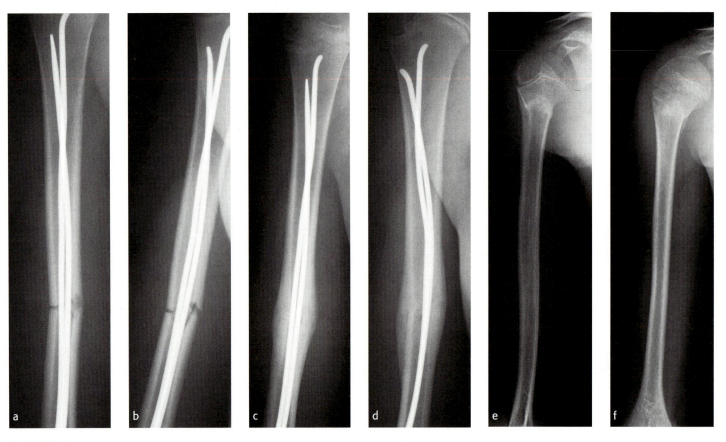

Fig 2.4-5a–f
a–b Postoperative AP and lateral x-rays demonstrate a good fracture reduction. There is wide separation of the bending apices at the fracture site.
c–d AP and lateral x-rays at 3 months postoperatively demonstrate full consolidation; nail removal is planned.
e–f AP and lateral x-rays taken 1 year after surgery; the child had a second (subcapital) humeral fracture showing completely remodeling of the previous fracture region.

2.4 Humeral shaft fracture, transverse, displaced (12-D/4.1)

5 Pitfalls –

Approach

Fig 2.4-6a–b Asymmetrical entrance sites and symmetric implantation can result in insufficient alignment because of the asymmetrical locations of the tension bands.

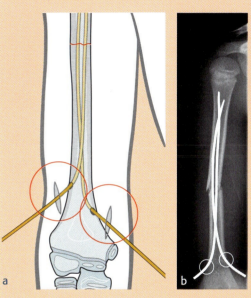

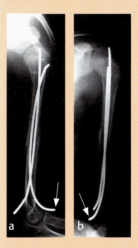

Fig 2.4-7a–b Nerve irritation.
a In the lateral approach, anterior or too anterior introduction of the nail can injure the radial nerve.
b On the medial side, too anterior or too posterior introduction of the nail can injure the median or ulnar nerve.

6 Pearls +

Approach

Fig 2.4-8 To obtain optimal alignment, the skin incisions along with the cortical holes must be exactly symmetrical.

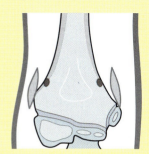

It is important to use the epicondyles as the reference points for the incisions. Palpate the lateral/medial edge of the humerus exactly and drill with care.

5 Pitfalls – (cont)

Reduction and fixation

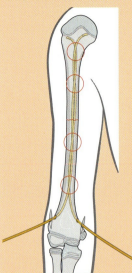

Fig 2.4-9 Twisting one nail around the other (corkscrew effect) compromises the bracing function of the nails and reduces the elasticity of the method. This results in an impairment of the stability of the reduction.

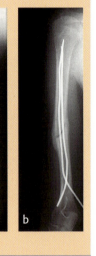

Fig 2.4-10a–b If a number of manipulations are necessary to introduce the nail into the second fragment, the shape of the nail may be visibly destroyed. Thus the tension bands are lost and no longer stabilize the fracture adequately.

Rehabilitation
Flexion and extension of the elbow may be limited if the ends of the nails irritate the fascia and the subcutaneous tissue.

6 Pearls + (cont)

Reduction and fixation
If during implantation and reduction a nail is rotated, it must be derotated to return the tip to its initial position. Avoid more than 180° turns.

If the nails become twisted, pull out one nail and reinsert another one.

This nail, which has lost its original tension band, needs to be changed to a new one with the correct mechanical properties.

Rehabilitation
Carefully cut the nails sufficiently so they will not irritate the subcutaneous tissues once active motion is begun. Avoid painful passive mobilization prior to nail removal. Occasionally, the nail end may need to be shortened to allow the resumption of free elbow motion.

3 Elbow

3.1 Introduction—elbow fractures 45
1 Indication 45
2 Patient preparation and positioning 46
3 Surgical principles 48
4 Postoperative care and implant removal 48

3.2 Supracondylar humeral fracture, closed, extension type (13-M/4.1–IV) 53

3.3 Supracondylar humeral fracture (13-M/4.1–IV) 59

3.4 Radial neck fracture, displaced (21-M/4.1-III) 63

3.5 Radial neck fracture, completely dislocated (21-E/2.1-III) 67

3.1 Introduction—elbow fractures

1 Indication

1.1 Supracondylar humeral fractures

Supracondylar humeral fractures are classified as 13-M/4 according to the AO comprehensive classification for long-bone fractures in children (see appendix).

There are four grades of displacement:
- I   undisplaced, no torsional failure
- II   displacement usually in the sagittal plane (antecurvature or recurvature), no torsional failure
- III additional displacement in a second, usually the coronal plane (antecurvature or recurvature and varus or valgus), torsional failure
- IV displacement in three planes or complete displacement without any fragment contact, torsional failure

Treatment based on classification

The principal treatment modality is usually based upon the exact classification:

Grade I: orthopedic treatment with plaster cast
Grade II:
- Gradual reduction by the Blount method (cuff and collar)
- Active manipulative reduction and immobilization with the Blount collar and cuff
- In some cases osteosynthesis will be necessary because the reduction cannot be adequately stabilized

Grades III/IV: reduction and surgical stabilization are necessary using the three common surgical techniques: percutaneous pinning, external radial fixator, or antegrade stabilization by ESIN.

Special indications

There are other conditions in which supracondylar fractures may need to be stabilized surgically:
- Those with flexion patterns
- Open fractures
- Those requiring vascular repair
- Patients with other major injuries (polytrauma)

In all cases needing reduction and fixation, ESIN is an option. Crossed percutaneous K-wire fixation following closed reduction is the most practiced method. However, it requires an additional cast and is associated with the risk of ulnar nerve injury (in case of bilateral crossed K-wires). Utilizing either an external fixator or ESIN allows early posttraumatic movement which may prevent some posttraumatic stiffness of the elbow. Intramedullary fixation has the lowest risk of a nerve injury occurring intraoperatively.

■■   Advantages
Only if perfect reduction is possible, ESIN has the following advantages over other methods of fixation:
- Excellent stability, hence no cast is necessary.
- The incidence of cubitus varus or cubitus valgus is very low.
- No implant crosses the elbow joint.

3 Elbow

1 Indication (cont)

1.2 Radial neck fractures

Indications
Radial neck fractures are classified as 21-M/1 or M/4 (see Appendix).

There are three grades of displacement:
I   no angulation and no displacement
II angulation with displacement less than half of the bone diameter
III angulation with displacement more than half of the bone diameter

Grade II and III fracture patterns usually require surgical intervention using one of the following two procedures: percutaneous manipulation and pinning, using the ESIN technique or the joystick technique.

Special indications
In children who have sustained a polytrauma, an ipsilateral fracture, or an injury in the extremity, the ESIN technique is especially useful as it eliminates the need for postoperative immobilization.
Because of the small potential for remodeling, a more precise anatomical reduction needs to be obtained with the ESIN technique in the child.

Advantages
There are four main advantages of the ESIN technique in the management of radial neck fractures:
- Because it avoids a direct approach to the fracture site, there is usually less trauma to the local vascular supply. This decreases the risk of avascular necrosis of the radial head.
- This technique avoids the need for transarticular fixation.
- The stability of the fixation is excellent which allows functional postoperative management.
- The use of postoperative immobilization in the form of a cast is usually not necessary.

2 Patient preparation and positioning

2.1 Supracondylar humeral fractures

Patient preparation
There is no international agreement as to whether displaced supracondylar humeral fractures need emergency intervention if there is no neurovascular damage. Often, the child's pain, the enormous swelling of the elbow and the impressive displacement of the fragment as seen on the x-rays will stimulate the surgeon to proceed with early operative intervention in these severely displaced fractures.

Medication
Antibiotic prophylaxis is indicated for open fractures. Their use with closed fractures should be managed according to the clinic protocol. Thrombosis prophylaxis is necessary only in generalized conditions associated with an elevated risk of intravascular clotting which are seldom seen in the pediatric age group. Some of the indications would be adolescent patients who are overweight, those who use tobacco products or use hormonal contraceptive drugs.

Patient positioning
The patient is placed in supine position with the injured upper limb on an arm table. The lateral translation of the patient requires an adaptive support for the head placed on the side of the table (Fig 3.1-1). The whole arm including the shoulder is surgically prepped and draped (Fig 3.1-2). Sterile drapes are needed to cover the image intensifier(s).

3.1 Introduction—elbow fractures

2 Patient preparation and positioning (cont)

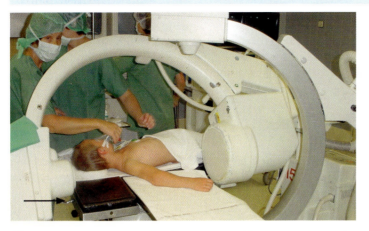 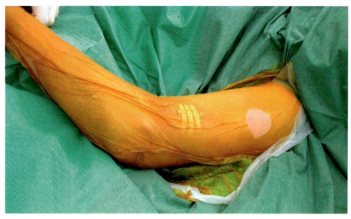

Fig 3.1-1 The patient is placed on the standard operating table with an attached radiolucent arm table. Since the child's head will need to be shifted laterally to facilitate visualization of the entire upper extremity, a separate support needs to be added (arrow). If available a second image intensifier may be helpful.

Fig 3.1-2 Patient draping. The entire upper extremity is prepped and draped, leaving only an opening in the stockingnette for the entrance site incisions.

Equipment
In addition to the basic orthopedic instruments, additional specialized instruments are needed to stabilize the fractures by the ESIN technique. These include:
- Standard ESIN set
- Nails:
  - 1.5–2.5 mm diameter, stainless steel, or titanium
  - The tip must be sharpened to facilitate penetration into the distal fragment
- K-wires can be useful as well
- Image intensifier. Normally, the AP view is easily achieved without changing the position of the intensifier. If two intensifiers are available, the procedure can be performed faster and more easily because the AP and lateral views can be obtained at the same time. This avoids rotation of the limb and/or image intensifier.

2.2 Radial neck fractures

Medication
The use of prophylactic antibiotics is based on the standards and guidelines of the clinic protocol.

Patient positioning
The patient is placed in the supine position with the affected upper limb on an arm table or directly on the reception surface of the intensifier. This latter position produces better imaging quality.

After positioning, the extremity is surgically prepped and draped free in a sterile fashion.

3 Elbow

2 Patient preparation and positioning   (cont)

Equipment
- In addition to the basic surgical instruments, the standard ESIN set including both the instruments and nails must be available.
- Only one image intensifier (C-arm) is necessary.
- Nails:
  1.5–2.5 mm diameter, stainless steel, or titanium; the selected nail should be 33% (1/3) of the diameter of the intramedullary canal.
- Sharpening of the tip of the nail is optional.

3 Surgical principles

3.1 Supracondylar humeral fractures

Surgical approaches
If a closed reduction cannot be accomplished, then an open reduction will be necessary. There is no agreement as to the best surgical approach. Some surgeons prefer to use a posterior incision, splitting the triceps muscle to expose the posterior aspect of the humerus and the fracture site. Others prefer to use a lateral and/or medial approach depending on where the suspected interposed tissue lies. Because the soft-tissue damage by the initial trauma is greatest anterior to the fracture, an anterior approach is preferred by many even in cases without vascular problems. This approach prevents additional soft-tissue trauma to the intact tissue posteriorly.

Methods of stabilization
Independent of the surgical approach chosen, the method of stabilization usually does not depend on the manner in which the fracture is reduced. K-wires can be used with either an open or closed reduction. An external fixator is easy to place following an open reduction. One advantage of the use of an external fixator is that by using the Schanz screws as joysticks to manipulate the fragments, a closed reduction may be facilitated. The ESIN technique of approaching the fracture in an antegrade manner can achieve a perfect and stable fixation as the ideal closed reduction. If the fracture site must be opened to achieve a satisfactory reduction, it is very easy to push the nails into both condyles by direct visualization. There is no evidence that any method of stabilization has any advantages over the other following an open reduction.

Direction of nailing
The nails are inserted in antegrade technique from a subdeltoid lateral incision using two different entrance sites.

3.2 Radial neck fractures

The standard retrograde approach starting distally in the radius as described in case 4.3 Forearm shaft fractures, transverse, is used.

4 Postoperative care and implant removal

4.1 Supracondylar humeral fractures

Postoperative x-ray inspection should be done in the operating room. No additional immobilization is necessary. Sometimes a sling is preferred for a few days for the safety of an anxious child. Movement is encouraged immediately, depending on the patient's level of comfort. Motion includes elbow flexion and extension in addition to pronation and supination of the forearm. Physiotherapy should be avoided during this phase. The patient is usually discharged from the hospital 24–48 hours postoperatively.

Outpatient follow-up
A follow-up x-ray 4–5 weeks after the initial surgery usually confirms sufficient callus formation. At this point, more active mobilization including sports activities can be permitted. By 2 to 3 months postoperatively, there should be full consolidation and remodeling visible on the x-rays prior to implant removal.

3.1 Introduction—elbow fractures

4 Postoperative care and implant removal (cont)

Implant removal
The implants are usually removed as an outpatient procedure. The standard ESIN set or flat-nosed pliers are necessary to remove the two nails.

4.2 Radial neck fractures

The first postoperative x-ray is obtained while still in the operating room. Postoperative additional immobilization is usually not necessary because of the stability achieved by this technique. Full early mobility is encouraged. A sling may be used for comfort and subjective safety. The patient is discharged 24–48 hours postoperatively. The first outpatient x-ray is obtained 4–5 weeks after discharge.

Rehabilitation
No special rehabilitation is required. Physiotherapy may be used in case of stiffness of the elbow. The mobility that is encouraged during the first weeks is limited to pronation and supination of the forearm. 3 weeks later, flexion and extension of the elbow are allowed in order to obtain a full range of motion.

Implant removal
The extracting pliers from the standard ESIN set, or, alternatively, flat-nosed pliers can be used to extract the nails.

Supracondylar humeral fractures

Pitfalls –	Pearls +
Approach Sometimes it is difficult to make the holes with the awl in the strong lateral cortex just below the deltoid muscle insertion. Injury to the radial nerve is possible if the drill slips at the posterior aspect of the humeral shaft. The first nail may be difficult to advance in the intramedullary canal because of the prebent tip. It may be difficult to introduce and advance the second nail antegrade easily. The nails cannot be advanced into the medial or lateral humeral columns.	**Approach** One option is to use a drill to make the entrance sites. It is important to drill the sites separately so that one is more proximal than the other. The humeral diaphysis should be held firmly between the surgeon's thumb and index finger when drilling the holes. During the drilling process the awl is directed from posterolateral toward anteromedial. The bent tip of the nail may need to be straightened. The first nail, which is inserted into the proximal entrance site, must be oriented toward the lateral humeral column The second nail must be advanced by alternating clockwise and counterclockwise rotatory movements so that it does not twist around the first nail. As it approaches the supracondylar area, it must be rotated 180° to direct it toward the medial humeral column.

Supracondylar humeral fractures   (cont)

Pitfalls –   (cont)

Reduction and fixation
The fracture cannot be reduced by a application of the usual external manipulative maneuvers.

The reduction of the fracture is not perfect.

Varus or a valgus alignment is observed.

Fig 3-1.3a–b   When a nail is advanced distally into the condyle, it penetrates the cortex of the distal fragment. The intramedullary nails do not fit correctly in the distal fragment but brake out dorsally, leading to a flexion failure and making revision necessary.

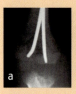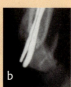

The distal fragment displaces as the nails are advanced.

Rehabilitation
Stiffness of the elbow.

Pearls +   (cont)

Reduction and fixation
The brachial muscle may occasionally become entrapped at the fracture site. In this rare occasion, an open reduction will be required.

Usually, the distal fragment is rotated in a medial direction. If this is the case, the proximal fragment, with the nails lying in its intramedullary canal, must likewise be rotated in a medial direction.

With this technique, the alignment of Baumann's angle in the distal fragment is easily visualized on the AP x-ray, as the elbow is not in hyperflexion.

As the nails are advanced into the distal humeral metaphysis, the direction of their tips must be very carefully monitored on both the AP and lateral x-ray images. At this point, the fracture must be perfectly reduced and stabilized by the surgeon so that the nail can be advanced with a hammer.

Sharp tips are essential to prevent distal fragment displacement. Reciprocal pressure on the olecranon or hyperflexion of the elbow can also be helpful.

Rehabilitation
Physiotherapy is optional but should not be initiated until at least 3 months after the initial trauma. If it is started during the acute phase, heterotopic ossification may be induced. Self-controlled spontaneous active mobilization by the patient alone will prevent most of the potential stiffness.

3.1 Introduction—elbow fractures

Radial neck fractures

Pitfalls –	Pearls +

Approach

The sensory branch of the radial nerve can be injured when making the entrance site in the distal radius.

The radial artery can be injured at the wrist.

The nail may be difficult to advance into the medullary canal of the radius.

Approach

The risk of injury can be lessened by the use of a transverse skin incision which is placed anterior to the lateral edge of the distal radial metaphysis. In addition, the use of a tourniquet and a larger surgical approach with dissection of the nerve may be helpful.

These problems can almost be eliminated by using a drill or a square-tipped awl to create the entrance site into the cortex in a posteromedial direction. The distal radius needs to be held firmly between the surgeon's thumb and index finger.

The tip of the nail is contoured enough to be advanced into the medullary canal. It is important that the tip is not contoured too much. This can cause an obstruction within the radius.

Reduction and fixation

Fig 3.1-4 A satisfactory reduction is not achieved with the nail using the joystick technique.

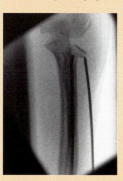

Reduction and fixation

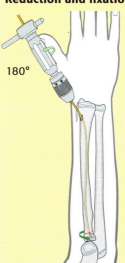

Fig 3.1-5 Reduce the head partially by rotating the nail. Then, remove the same nail from the proximal epiphysis, rotate it 180°, and advance it again into the epiphysis. This new rotation maneuver should lead to the final reduction of the fracture.

Radial neck fractures (cont)

Pitfalls – (cont)

Reduction and fixation (cont)
The radial head may be very thin, making it difficult to stabilize with the nail tip.

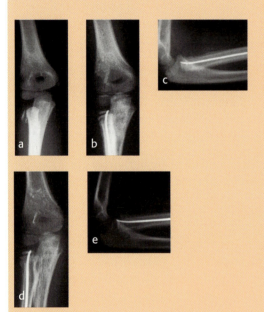

Fig 3.1-6a–e For stabilization of a very small radial head fragment, especially in younger children, the physis must be penetrated.
a   Injury x-ray with complete displaced radial head.
b–c Situation after closed reduction with "joystick" technique.
d–e Healing without sign of necrosis after 2 months.

Rehabilitation
Stiffness of the elbow is rare.

Pearls + (cont)

Reduction and fixation (cont)
Fig 3.1-7a–e Alternatively a K-wire can be used percutaneously as a joystick to force the head into a satisfactory position. To avoid injury to the radial nerve, this K-wire is introduced through the lateral part of the proximal forearm in full pronation. Thus, the radial nerve is shifted in an anterior direction and away from the K-wire.

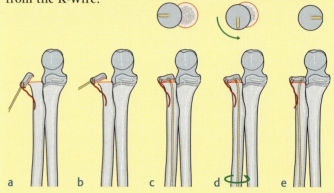

Open reduction. If closed has not been achieved by any of the previous techniques, an open reduction must be performed using a posterolateral approach. Often only a small flap of periosteum is attached at the radial head. If it is destroyed the risk of avascular necrosis is relevant. Therefore reduction without an incision of the articular capsule (open, but transcapsular manipulation) may be an option to save the periosteal blood supply.

In young patients, with a very small radial head, a plaster cast must be worn for 3–4 weeks.

Rehabilitation
Gentle active physiotherapy against resistance can be ordered.

3.2 Supracondylar humeral fracture, closed, extension type (13-M/4.1-IV)

1 Case description

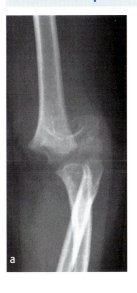
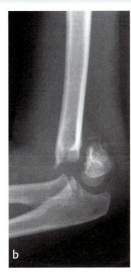

A 5-year-old girl jumped from a climbing frame and fell, using her right upper extremity with the elbow extended to break her fall. She presented to the hospital with visible displacement and significant swelling in the supracondylar area. Her neurovascular function was normal. The x-rays showed a fully displaced distal humeral fracture (Fig 3.2-1). She was transferred immediately to the operating room because of the marked displacement of the fracture fragments. This was done even though emergency intervention is usually only necessary in those cases with a pulseless white forearm and hand.

Fig 3.2-1a–b   Preoperative x-rays. AP and lateral views demonstrating a type IV posterolateral supracondylar fracture pattern of the right distal humerus.

2 Surgical approach

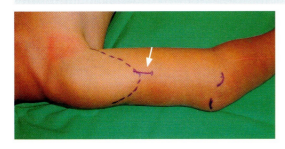

Fig 3.2-2   The skin incision (arrow) for the entry points is made on the lateral aspect of the middle third of the arm just below the humeral insertion of the deltoid muscle (dotted line).

An initial reduction of the fracture should always be performed prior to the sterile draping of the extremity. With general and additional plexus anesthesia, a preliminary reduction is obtained. Initially, gentle axial traction is applied along the axis of the forearm with countertraction at the humerus. Once the length has been reestablished, the elbow is flexed as the thumb of the surgeon simultaneously pushes forward on the olecranon.

C-arm control
Control the quality of the reduction in the coronal plane using the AP image intensifier views. A Baumann's angle between 70° and 80° must be achieved. Control the quality of the reduction in the sagittal plane with the lateral C-arm control views. The angle of the shaft to the condyles of the humeral distal epiphysis (shaft–condylar angle) needs to be reduced to between 30° and 40°.

Skin incision
The skin is incised for a distance of 4 cm on the lateral side of the arm from the midthird proximally to just below the distal insertion of the deltoid muscle (Fig 3.2-2).

2 Surgical approach (cont)

Approach
The subcutaneous tissue is dissected until the lateral cortex of the humerus is reached. The periosteum is incised. The lateral cortex is perforated with an awl. Initially, it is drilled at right angles to prevent the tip from slipping. Once the cortex has been penetrated, the awl handle is angled 45° to the shaft axis to produce an oblique canal. This facilitates the introduction of the nails into the medullary canal (Fig 3.2-3). Two sites are required with one being more proximal and the second slightly more anterior and distal than the other.

Nail advancement
The two nails are not precontoured, but their tips are bent and sharpened. As they are introduced and advanced antegrade into the diaphysis, the tips are directed towards the lateral cortex (Fig 3.2-4).

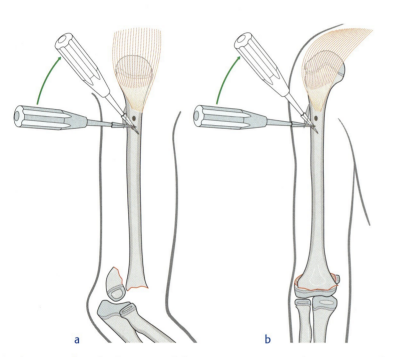

Fig 3.2-3a–b   The location of the entrance sites on the proximal humerus.
a   Lateral view.
b   AP view.

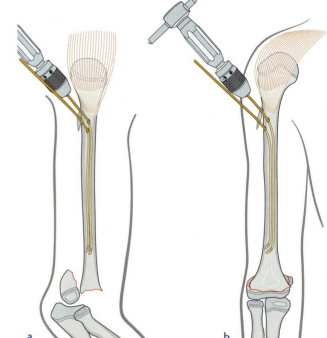

Fig 3.2-4a–b   Distal advancement. The nails are advanced antegrade to the fracture. At this point the tips of both nails are pointing laterally.
a   Lateral view.
b   AP view.

3.2 Supracondylar humeral fracture, closed, extension type (13-M/4.1-IV)

2 Surgical approach (cont)

When the tips are being advanced into the metaphysis, the more distally implanted nail is rotated 180° toward the medial column (Fig 3.2-5). This needs to be accomplished carefully to prevent one nail from twisting totally around the other nail. The tip of the most proximally inserted nail remains directed laterally. In the lateral view, the tips of both nails are turned slightly so that they are pointing directly toward the metaphysis.

3 Reduction and fixation

Reduction
The fracture is again reduced as previously described under the control of a C-arm. The elbow may be flexed to 60° to obtain a better AP view as long as the reduction is perfect on the lateral view (Fig 3.2-6).

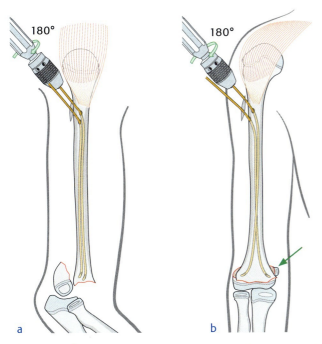

Fig 3.2-5a–b Nail rotation. As the nails are entering the metaphysis, the tip of the most distally inserted nail is rotated 180° so that it advances into the medial column (arrow).
a Lateral view.
b AP view.

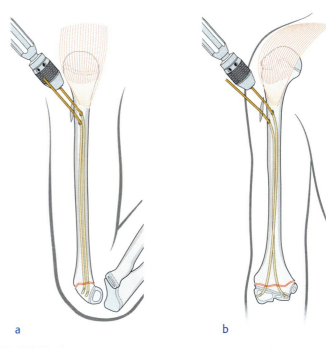

Fig 3.2-6a–b Reduction and stabilization. The fracture fragments are stabilized with flexion of the elbow. Once reduced, the tips of the nails are then carefully advanced into the distal fragment.
a Lateral view.
b AP view.

3 Reduction and fixation (cont)

Stabilization

The reduction is maintained by the surgeon while an assistant advances the nails one at a time by gentle hammer blows as far as a few millimeters proximal to the fracture line. Rotation of the nails must be strictly avoided during this maneuver. Progression of the nails into the distal humerus is controlled under the C-arm (Fig 3.2-7). If both implants are reliably introduced into the distal fragment, the nails can be impacted into the distal metaphyseal bone (Fig. 3.2-8). The proximal part of each nails is cut so that it lies under the skin. Closure of the skin is accomplished in the standard manner.

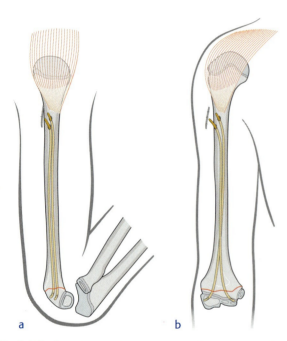
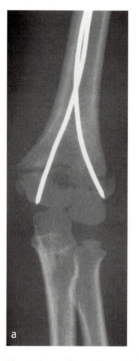
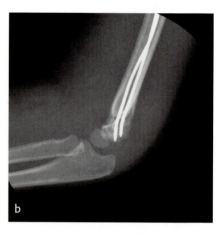

Fig 3.2-7a–b Final nail insertion. The proximal ends of the nails are cut and inserted to be flush with the cortex. The incisions are closed.
a   Lateral view.
b   AP view.

Fig 3.2-8a–b AP and lateral postoperative x-rays demonstrating the anatomical reduction and fixation with the tips impacted in the metaphysis. On the AP view, the Baumann's angle is normal. On the lateral view, the shaft–condylar angle has been restored. This provides sufficient stabilization to permit full postoperative mobilization.

3.2 Supracondylar humeral fracture, closed, extension type (13-M/4.1-IV)

4 Postoperative care and rehabilitation

The use of a sling to ameliorate pain at the upper extremity is optional for a few days. A cast is not necessary. Physiotherapy is not recommended. Movement of the arm is not limited except by pain.

Nails are usually removed after 2 months, depending on the consolidation of the bone (Fig 3.2-9). One month later, the patient was fully active without any functional restrictions.

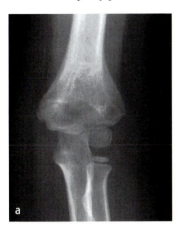
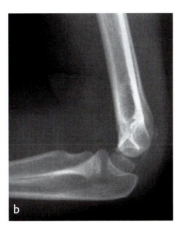

Fig 3.2-9a–b   Full recovery. AP and lateral x-rays taken after nail removal. A complete anatomical and functional recovery has been achieved.

5 Pitfalls –

Approach
If the entrance canals are perpendicular to the bone axis, it is difficult to introduce the nails.

The tip of one nail cannot be placed in the aimed condylar column.

Reduction and fixation
Because of friction it may be difficult to advance the second nail distally. Rotation of the nail may be necessary to advance it.

6 Pearls +

Approach
Obliquity of the holes toward the elbow makes the progression of the nails easier.

Sometime it is helpful to "change the side": The proximal nail may more easily be placed in the medial column and the distal nail in the lateral column.

Reduction and fixation
As the second nail is advanced, care must be taken to avoid twisting it around the first nail which can create a corkscrew phenomenon. The nail needs to be rotated alternately clockwise and counterclockwise rather than making a complete rotation.

5 Pitfalls − (cont)

Reduction and fixation   (cont)
The nails may penetrate the cortex of the distal metaphysis and end up in the joint cavity.

6 Pearls +   (cont)

Reduction and fixation   (cont)
Rotation maneuvers are not carried out when crossing the fracture line. Withdraw the nails proximally a few millimeters to again orient the tips exactly and then advance the nails again in a distal direction.

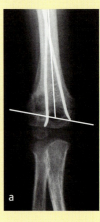
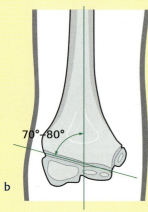

Fig 3.2-10a–b   It is important that the Baumann's angle on the AP view measures between 70° and 80°.

3.3 Supracondylar humeral fracture (13-M/4.1–IV)

1 Case description

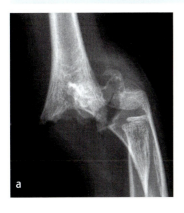
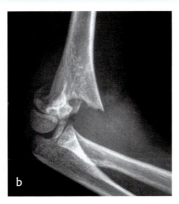

A 10-year-old boy sustained an injury to his left upper extremity while doing a judo maneuver. He presented to the emergency room with a deformed and swollen left elbow. A clinical examination revealed an absent radial pulse with absent function of both the radial nerve and the anterior interosseous branch of the median nerve. The initial x-rays revealed a type IV supracondylar extension fracture pattern with posterolateral displacement of the distal fragment (Fig 3.3-1).

Fig 3.3-1a–b X-rays of the left elbow taken on arrival at the emergency room. A type IV extension fracture pattern with a posterolaterally displaced distal fragment.

2 Surgical approach

The surgical approach that is required for this case has been described in detail in chapter 3.2 Supracondylar humeral fracture, closed, extension type.

The most important aspect in the management of this patient is the return of the radial pulse after preliminary reduction.

3 Reduction and fixation

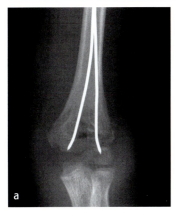
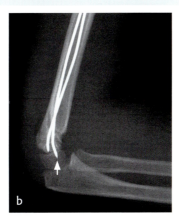

Physeal penetration
Nails of 2.0 mm or K-wires of 1.8 mm diameter are best for this type of fracture. The reduction and fixation were performed exactly as described in the previous case.
Because the distal fragment is very small, the radial nail will need to perforate the physis of the lateral condyle in this case. The tip must be secured deep inside the capitulum (Fig 3.3-2).

Experience in many prior cases has shown that there are no growth consequences from penetration of the physes with the smooth nails. It must be emphasized at this point that multiple perforations of the physis or vigorous rotation of the nail tip during the advancement process must be avoided.

Fig 3.3-2a–b Postreduction x-rays. AP and lateral x-rays following stabilization using the ESIN antegrade technique. Because the distal fragment was so small, the tip of the lateral nail was rotated anteriorly to penetrate the physis to provide more stable seating in the epiphysis of the lateral condyle (arrow).

4 Postoperative care and rehabilitation

Early motion
The use of a cast or sling is not recommended. The stability of the nails within the capitulum allows early mobilization and intensive physiotherapy for rehabilitation. With this patient, physiotherapy was prescribed for rehabilitation of the radial and interosseous nerve palsies. Both nerves demonstrated full recovery within 2 weeks.

2 weeks postoperatively, the patient had flexion to 100° and extension to 70°. By 6 weeks, elbow flexion had increased to 130° with extension progressing to 30°.

Follow-up and implant removal
X-rays obtained 3 months postoperatively demonstrated a normal anatomical alignment with good fixation. On the AP view the Baumann's angle is 80°. On the lateral view, the shaft–condylar angle is 30°. Fracture healing was complete, thus permitting nail removal (Fig 3.3-3).

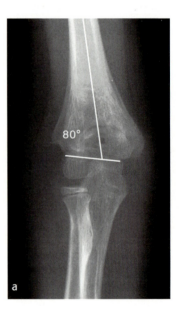
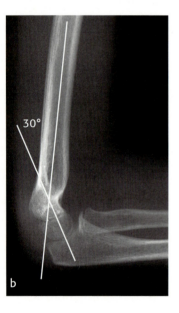

Fig. 3.3-3a–b AP and lateral x-rays taken following nail removal demonstrate anatomical alignment of the distal fragment along with complete healing of the fracture. There seems to be no growth disturbance of the lateral condylar physis due to the penetration of the nail.

3.3 Supracondylar humeral fracture (13-M/4.1–IV)

5 Pitfalls –

Reduction and fixation
Even though the radial pulse is restored, the fracture cannot be reduced by manipulative methods alone. This is usually the result of muscle interposition or because the tip of a fragment is buttonholed into the surrounding soft tissues.

The fracture line is very distal. This makes it difficult to obtain sufficient fixation within the small distal metaphysis.

6 Pearls +

Reduction and fixation
Open reduction is necessary. One of the standard surgical approaches (posterior, anterior, medial, or lateral) is used according to the type of fracture and the surgeon's preference Open reduction is not a contradiction to the use of ESIN. Following an open reduction, there is a higher incidence of scarring of the joint capsule and other soft-tissue structures at the elbow. The possibility of immediate postoperative mobilization makes the ESIN method especially attractive.

Positioning of both nail tips anteriorly allows them to be advanced more distally. This results in a more stable fixation. The physis can be penetrated by the smooth tip of the nail with little risk of growth arrest (see Fig 3.3-3).

3 Elbow

3.4 Radial neck fracture, displaced (21-M/4.1-III)

1 Case description

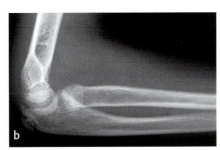

Fig 3.4-1a–b Primary reduction. AP and lateral x-rays of the left elbow following an attempt at conservative management reveal an unsatisfactory alignment of the radial head in relation to the proximal shaft.

Following a fall on his outstretched upper extremity, this 9-year-old boy presented to the hospital with pain and swelling localized in the left proximal forearm. X-rays revealed a displaced radial neck fracture.

After adequate relaxation was achieved with general anesthesia, an attempt to reduce the fracture by conservative management was first made by applying gentle axial traction on the forearm. Following this, the surgeon applied pressure directly over the radial head with the elbow flexed. At the same time, the forearm was forced into full pronation. Images obtained on the C-arm following this conservative procedure, revealed an incomplete reduction (Fig 3.4-1).

■■ It is always important that attempts at closed reduction are performed prior to surgically prepping and draping of the injured extremity.

2 Surgical approach

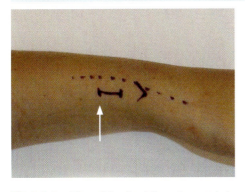

Fig 3.4-2 The skin incision (arrow) is located proximal to the radial styloid (oblique line). It must also lie anterior to the superficial radial nerve (dotted line).

Skin incision
A 2 cm long skin incision is made at the lateral aspect of the distal forearm just proximal to the distal physis of the radius (Fig 3.4-2). It is very important that the incision is palmar to the superficial branch of the radial nerve and the superficial radial vein. An alternative approach is to make the incision dorsally to create the entrance site in the dorsal cortex through the palpable dorsal tubercle of radius as described in case 4.3 Forearm shaft fracture, transverse (see Fig 4.3-3).

Approach
The subcutaneous tissue is dissected to the lateral cortex of the radius. The periosteum is incised. Next, the lateral cortex is perforated to create the entrance site with either the square tipped awl or using a 3–3.5 mm drill. It is important that the drill is perpendicular to the cortex until it is well seated in the bone. This prevents the drill from slipping off the cortex. Only a single entrance site is needed.

2 Surgical approach (cont)

Advancement of the nails

The nail is introduced through the entrance site and is advanced retrograde into the radial diaphysis (Fig 3.4-3a). It may be necessary to rotate the tip once or twice. The surgeon also needs to understand that when the sharp tip of the nail reaches the radial head, it needs to be positioned with the tip in the plane of the maximal head displacement (Fig 3.4-3b).

3 Reduction and fixation

Reduction

Under C-arm control an indirect reduction of the radial head is achieved by the surgeon using the thumb to apply direct pressure over the head fragment (Fig 3.4-4a). Then, the assistant surgeon uses the hammer to gently advance the nail tip into the head. Rotation of the nail must be strictly avoided during this maneuver in order not to avoid creating a cavity in the center of the metaphysis. At this point, the radial head is secured by the nail tip. The final reduction can be achieved by gently rotating the nail with the T-handle as the forearm is rotated into pronation (Fig 3.4-4b). During this process, direct pressure is

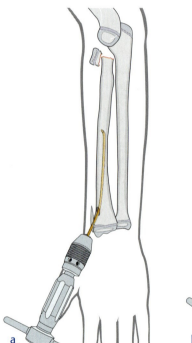
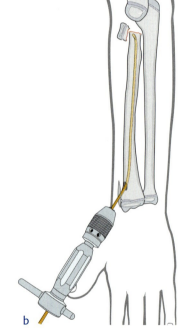

Fig 3.4-3a–b
a Diaphyseal insertion.
   After passing through the distal metaphyseal entrance site, the nail is advanced retrograde into the diaphysis.
b Radial head entrance.
   When the nail tip exits the neck, the tip is directed to the radial head.

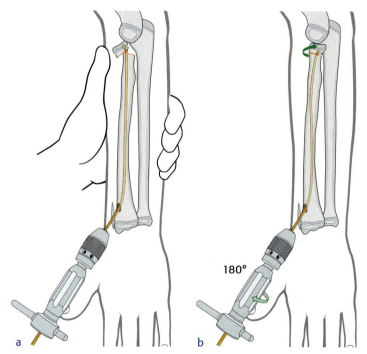

Fig 3.4-4a–b
a Indirect reduction.
   Once the tip is directed toward the center of the head, direct manual pressure is applied to the head fragment to achieve partial reduction.
b Nail rotation.
   When the tip is secured within the head fragment, the final reduction is achieved by rotating the nail (arrow).

3.4 Radial neck fracture, displaced (21-M/4.1-III)

3 Reduction and fixation   (cont)

applied to the lateral part of the radial head. Reduction must be carried out at all times under C-arm control.

Final seating
Once the surgeon is satisfied with the final reduction, the nail is secured by impacting the tip to penetrate the physis of the radial head. This places the tip just within the subchondral bone of the epiphysis (Fig 3.4-5). After final seating has been achieved, the distal part of the nail is bent 90° and cut so that the tip lies deep below the skin (Fig 3.4-6).

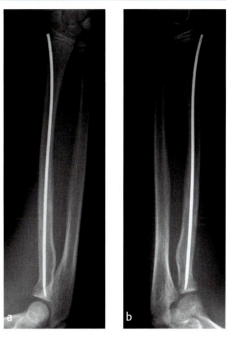

Fig 3.4-6a–b   Postoperative x-rays. The proximal end of the nail has been cut; the tip only just penetrates the physis.

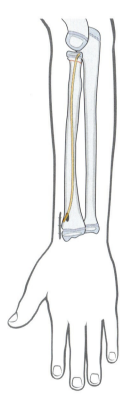

Fig 3.4-5   Final position.
The nail is in its final position with the head well aligned and reduced. The tip is fixed deep in the epiphysis.

4 Postoperative care and rehabilitation

Early functional recovery.

The only situation in which a cast is felt to be necessary is in the very young child with a thin epiphysis. Even then, it is not indicated for more than 3 weeks. As soon as postoperative pain permits, early active motion is encouraged.

The nails cannot be removed less than 8 weeks after surgery.

5 Pitfalls −

Approach
Damage of the superficial branch of the radial nerve or the radial artery.

Reduction and fixation
The nail is advanced by gentle hammer blows until it rests securely in the radial head. In this part of the stabilization process, rotation of the nail must be avoided as the tip will destroy the cancellous bone of the head. This in turn can create a cavity which will not provide adequate fixation.

To obtain the final reduction, the rotation of the nail must be gentle and performed in conjunction with the pronation of the forearm.

6 Pearls +

Approach
When creating the entrance site in the cortex, take care to avoid injury to the radial artery ensuring that the awl or drill does not slip in an anterior direction. Cranial obliquity of the entrance canals will greatly facilitate the retrograde advancement of the nails. Entry point through Lister's tubercle.

Reduction and fixation
If the reduction of the radial head is incomplete, it is often helpful to remove the nail from the epiphysis. It is then reoriented toward the lateral part of the head. Rotation of the nail to reduce the head into correct alignment is repeated.

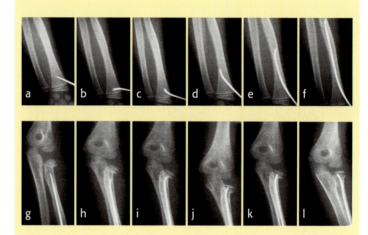

Fig 3.4-7a–l   The series of x-rays illustrates the reduction and fixation of the radial head in a descriptive way.

3.5 Radial neck fracture, completely dislocated (21-E/2.1-III)

1 Case description

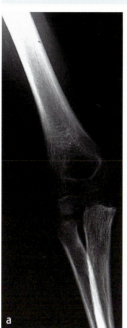

An 8-year-old girl used her right outstretched arm to break her fall. She presented with pain and swelling in the right elbow area. The injury x-rays (Fig 3.5-1) were interpreted as being normal. Because of failure to promptly resolve her symptoms, she was seen in another facility by a second surgeon who recognized the true nature of her injury. He determined that the radial head was completely dislocated. The true nature of this fracture was difficult to appreciate because the displacement of the radial head was complete, lying proximally in the adjacent soft tissues at 90° to the radial neck (Fig 3.5-2). A more careful evaluation of the image demonstrates that the head appeared like a disk on the AP image and the neck was subluxated posterolaterally in relationship to the capitulum.

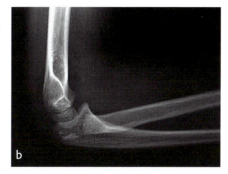
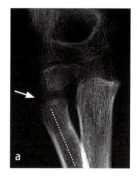
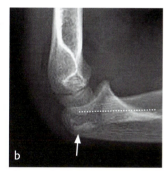

Fig 3.5-1a–b   Injury x-rays. These AP and lateral x-rays taken at the first hospital were interpreted as being normal.

Fig 3.5-2a–b   A closer look. On the AP view, the radial head has a disc-like appearance (arrow). The radial head is seen to be rotated by 90° to the proximal radius (arrow) on the lateral view. On both images, the proximal radius is not aligned with the center of the lateral condylar ossification (dotted line).

2 Surgical approach

Initially, an elastic nail was introduced into the radius using the distal lateral metaphyseal entrance point as described in chapter 3.1 Introduction—elbow fractures.

3 Reduction and fixation

Initial treatment
Initially, the exact position of the radial head fragment was not appreciated, subsequently, the standard ESIN technique was initiated. In the first procedure, which was performed under a general anesthesia, a satisfactory reduction was felt to have been obtained following a closed manipulative maneuver.

The standard 2.0 mm ESIN nail with an extremely sharp tip was used. The nail was introduced through the entrance site and advanced retrograde into the radial diaphysis. Once the fracture site had been reached, the tip was oriented in a lateral and posterior direction in anticipation of entering the head.

When the nail tip had reached the fracture site, a more careful examination of the images revealed that the radial head was "upside down" (Fig 3.5-3).

Open reduction
To reduce this fracture adequately, an open reduction was performed using the posterolateral approach. Once the head was visualized, it was found to be vascularized by only a very narrow flap of periosteum. With this degree of displacement the risk of avascular necrosis can be very high.

Final stabilization
The radial head was carefully and gently rotated around its thin pedicle in order to achieve perfect reduction. Once a satisfactory situation had been achieved, the nail tip was then advanced into the radial head to achieve excellent stability (Fig 3.5-4).

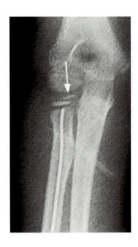

Fig 3.5-3 "Upside down". In this intraoperative image, the articular surface of the radial head is situated facing the fracture surface of the proximal fragment. A clue to this reverse positioning of the head is the metaphyseal fragment facing the articular surface of the capitulum (arrow).

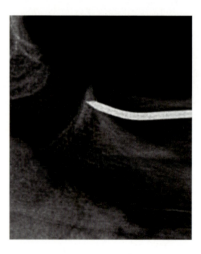

Fig 3.5-4 Final stabilization. In this lateral x-ray taken immediately postoperatively, the head is anatomically reduced with the tip of the nail lying in the subchondral area of the head fragment.

4 Postoperative care and rehabilitation

Because of the small size of the head fragment, there was concern about postoperative stability. Therefore, it was decided to place the extremity in a long-arm plaster cast for 6 weeks. The family was also informed of the possibility that avascular necrosis of the radial head might develop.

3.5 Radial neck fracture, completely dislocated (21-E/2.1-III)

5 Pitfalls –

Reduction and fixation

Fig 3.5-5a–j   15-year-old female; fell off her bicycle and onto her outstretched arm.

a–b   The injury x-rays show a dislocation of the elbow joint with initially undisplaced radial neck fracture. Closed reduction was immediately performed under image intensifier control. At this point in time, the radial head was completely displaced posteriorly.

c–d   Open reduction was performed, fixation of the radial head with two nails to treat rotational instability. The postoperative x-ray shows persisting radial head dislocation.

e–f   Secondary intervention two days later; a bone block from the ulna was inserted as bone graft.

g–j   There were no signs of healing over the next three months, but also no signs of necrosis. The nail was removed. The mobility of the elbow is normal in the absence of fracture healing.

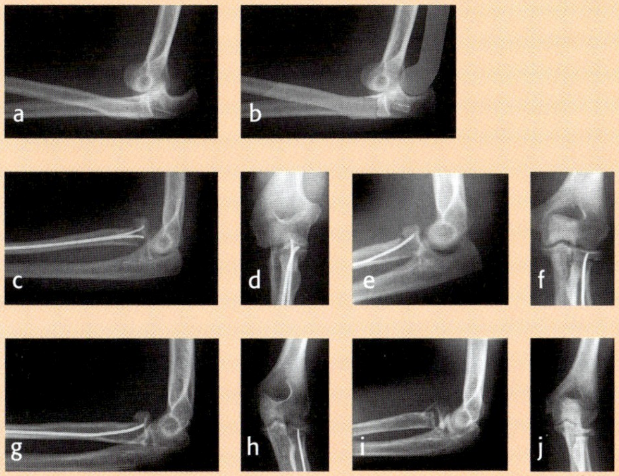

6 Pearls +

Reduction and fixation

Fig 3.5-6a–i   Completely displaced radial neck fracture in an 11-year-old girl. Closed, indirect reduction can be difficult. In this situation, transcutaneous manipulation of the radial head with a K-wire will be possible. With this so-called "joystick" technique the fragment can be manipulated in such a way that the fragment can later be engaged by the tip of the nail.

a–b   AP and lateral views of the fully displaced radial head.

c–d   The transcutaneously inserted K-wire pushes the radial head onto the metaphysis.

e–f   Intraoperative x-rays show perfect reduction and alignment.

g–h   Postoperative x-rays at 2 months show good healing. The child never needed an additional restraint plaster cast. Full mobility was achieved.

i   Care must be taken to ensure that the K-wire enters the radial head and does not exit through the fracture gap.

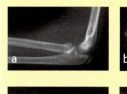
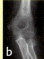
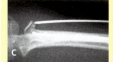

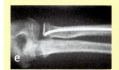
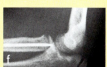
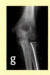
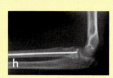
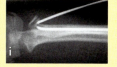

4 Forearm

4.1 **Introduction—forearm fractures** **71**
  1 Indication 71
  2 Patient preparation and positioning 72
  3 Surgical principles 73
  4 Implant removal 74
  5 Suggested reading 75

4.2 **Monteggia lesion (22-D/6.1)** **77**

4.3 **Forearm shaft fractures, transverse (12-D/4.1)** **81**

4.4 **Radial and ulnar shaft fractures, displaced radius with butterfly fragment, ulna simple (12-D/5.2)** **91**

4.5 **Radial and ulnar shaft fractures, malunion following conservative treatment (22-D/4.1)** **95**

4.6 **Radial and ulnar shaft refracture after conservative treatment (22-D/4.1)** **99**

4.7 **Distal radial and ulnar diaphyseal-metaphyseal fractures, displaced (22-D/4.1)** **103**

4.1 Introduction—forearm fractures

1 Indication

Many fractures of the radial and ulnar shafts are amenable to conservative management. However, many fracture patterns are better treated with ESIN stabilization. Any surgeon managing these fractures needs to be acquainted with the specific surgical indications. These are not dependent on the patient's age.

Specific indications
Some of the definite indications for surgical stabilization of radial and ulnar shaft fractures include:
- Complete fractures of both bones
  This is especially true if the fractures are on the same level, have oblique fracture planes, or a convergent displacement. The more proximal the fracture site, the greater the threshold to surgical stabilization.
- Greenstick fracture patterns
  Greenstick fractures of both shafts may require stabilization if reduction and stabilization with a cast does not achieve satisfactory alignment. This is especially critical if the residual angulation is greater than 10° since these fractures have a tendency to reangulate to their initial position.
- An isolated fracture of the radius
  Those isolated fractures with an irreducible valgus deviation of more than 10°, which cannot be corrected by a wedging of the cast, will need to be surgically stabilized.
- Monteggia lesions
  It is often difficult to obtain or maintain radial head reduction unless the ulna is anatomically reduced. This can be a problem particularly if there is radial bowing of the ulna.
- Distal fracture patterns
  In the transition zone of the distal metaphysis to diaphysis of the radius, ESIN is indicated only if the retrograde radial nail can reach the opposite inner cortex of the distal fragment before crossing the fracture line. Furthermore, antegrade nailing of the radius is NOT recommended because of the risk of injury to the deep branch of the radial nerve. Distal fractures of the ulna can easily be stabilized with the standard antegrade nailing approach.
- Refractures
  It is best to avoid treating these nonoperatively whenever possible. This is because repeated immobilization with a cast would only further weaken the upper extremity muscles that are already weak from the preceding period of immobilization.
- Ipsilateral humeral fractures
- Open fractures
- Polytrauma

4 Forearm

2 Patient preparation and positioning

These fractures should be treated as an emergency only if there is an open fracture, neurovascular injury, or imminent perforation of the skin.

Medication
With open fractures, antibiotic prophylaxis is definitely required. With closed fractures, antibiotics are administered according to the standards of the clinic protocol. Thrombosis prophylaxis is utilized only in those patients immobilized because of multiple injuries or other general diseases with risk factors such as obesity or those patients on contraceptive medication.

Patient positioning
The patient is placed supine with the arm on an arm table (Fig 4.1-1). If preferred, the fracture region can be placed directly on the C-arm receiver protected with a sterile cover. Using sterile technique the injured extremity is surgically prepped and draped to above the elbow. The hand may be covered with a glove.

Equipment
In addition to the basic orthopedic instruments, additional specialized instruments and implants are needed to apply the ESIN technique. These include:
- Standard ESIN set
- Nails:
  2.0–3.0 mm diameter stainless steel or titanium; each of the selected nails should be 2/3 the diameter of the radial and/or ulnar medullary canal at midshaft.
- Image intensifier:
  This should be set up in such a manner that it does not interfere with the surgical field. To be most effective, it must be positioned so that the surgeon has a direct view of the monitor.

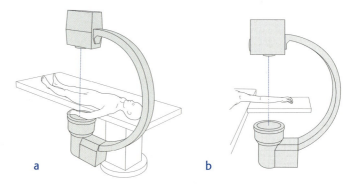

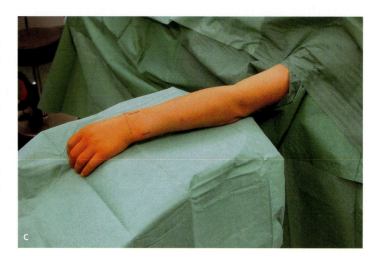

Fig 4.1-1a–c Patient positioning.
a–b Illustrations showing the positioning of the arm directly on the C-arm receiver or on an arm table.
c Correct placement of the forearm directly on the radiolucent arm-side extension. The patient has been placed as far laterally on the table as possible.

4.1 Introduction—forearm fractures

3 Surgical principles

There are three basic principles that need to be considered when using the ESIN technique in the management of fractures of the radial and ulnar shaft. These are:
1. The choice of nailing approaches.
2. The determination of the entrance sites.
3. The spreading of the interosseous membrane.

Nailing approaches
There are specific approaches available for nailing the radial and ulnar shafts.
1. Radius: retrograde nailing from a lateral or dorsal (radial tubercle) entrance site (Fig 4.1-2a–b) is the only technique utilized. It must be remembered that antegrade nailing of the radius is contraindicated.
2. Ulna: this can be achieved by one of the following two techniques:
   - Antegrade from the lateral cortex of the olecranon (Fig 4.1-2a–b).
   - Retrograde from the medial cortex of the distal metaphysis (Fig 4.1–2c).

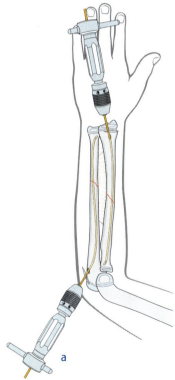
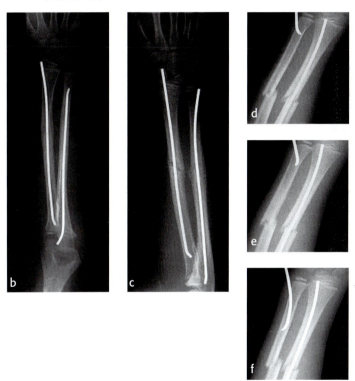

Fig 4.1-2a–f Nailing approaches.
a Retrograde nailing approach of the radius and antegrade approach of the ulna.
b X-ray demonstrating healing of shaft fractures following the use of a retrograde radial and an antegrade ulnar approach.
c X-ray demonstrating healing of shaft fractures following the use of retrograde approaches for both the radius and ulna.
d–f X-rays showing the process of a retrograde approach from the medial cortex of the distal metaphysis of the ulna.

3 Surgical principles (cont)

Entrance sites
The specific locations of the entrance sites for these approaches will be described later in the chapters dealing with each individual technique.

Interosseous spreading
The interosseous membrane is spread in an oval fashion by placing the nail tips in opposition so that they are facing each other (Fig 4.1-3). Thus, both bones are stabilized by recreating their physiological curve.

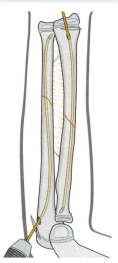

Fig 4.1-3   Interosseous spreading. Schematic drawing demonstrating spreading of the interosseous membrane by directing the nail tips toward each other.

4 Implant removal

3 months with the nails in place is sufficient in many cases.

By 3 months postinjury, the x-rays should show full consolidation with complete remodeling (Fig 4.1-4). At this point, nail removal can be performed as an outpatient procedure. If consolidation and remodeling are not complete, removal may be postponed for another month without reservation. Some authors do not recommend removal before 8 months postinjury because of the risk of refracture. In our experience, the refracture rate was not higher for those removed at 3 months. Significant skin irritation in the implantation area requiring premature removal has rarely been encountered.

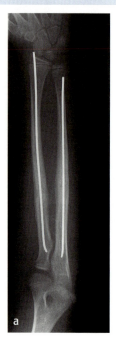 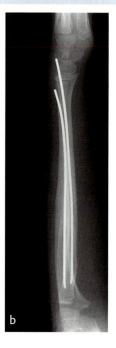

Fig 4.1-4a–b   AP and lateral x-rays taken 3 months following ESIN stabilization of this patient demonstrate consolidation and remodeling sufficient to permit nail removal. Note that these nails were both inserted via a retrograde approach.

4.1 Introduction—forearm fractures

5 Suggested reading

Aribit F, Laville JM (1999)
Postero-medial elastic stable intramedullary nailing for anteriorly displaced distal diaphyso-metaphyseal fractures of the radius in children.
Rev chir orthop; 85(8):858–860.

Fuller DJ, McCullough CJ (1982)
Malunited fractures of the forearm in children.
J Bone Joint Surg; 64(3):364–367.

Hahn MP, Richter D, Ostermann PAW, et al (1996)
[Elastic intramedullary nailing—a concept for the management of unstable forearm fractures in childhood.]
Chirurg; 67(4):409–412.

Knorr P, Dietz HG (1999)
Die elastisch stabile Markraumschienung bei Schaftfrakturen des Unterarms im Kindesalter–Indikationen, Technik, Ergebnisse.
Klin Pädiatr; 211:115.

Laer L, Hasler C (2000)
[Spontaneous corrections, growth disorders and posttraumatic deformities after fractures in the area of the forearm of the growing skeleton.]
Handchir Mikrochir Plast Chir; 32(4):231–241.

Lascombes P, Prevot J, Ligier JN, et al (1990)
Elastic stable intramedullary nailing in forearm shaft fractures in children: 85 cases.
J Pediatr Orthop; 10(2):167–171.

Lee S, Nicol RO, Stott NS (2002)
Intramedullary fixation for pediatric unstable forearm fractures.
Clin Orthop Relat Res; (402):245–250.

Lieber J, Joeris A, Knorr P, et al (2005)
ESIN in forearm fractures: clear indications often used, but some avoidable complications.
Eur J Trauma; 31(1):3–11.

Mann D, Schnabel M, Baacke M, et al (2003)
[Results of elastic stable intramedullary nailing (ESIN) in forearm fractures in childhood.]
Unfallchirurg; 106(2):102–109.

Matthews LS, Kaufer H, Garver DF, et al (1982)
The effect on supination-pronation of angular malalignment of fractures of both bones of the forearm.
J Bone Joint Surg Am; 64(1):14–17.

Ostermann PA, Richter D, Mecklenburg K, et al (1999)
[Pediatric forearm fractures: indications, technique, and limits of conservative management.]
Unfallchirurg; 102(10):784–790.

Parsch K (1990)
Die Morote-Drahtung bei proximalen und mittleren Unterarmschaftfrakturen des Kindes.
Operat Orthop Traumatol; 2:245–255.

Schmittenbecher PP, Dietz HG, Linhart WE, et al (2000)
Complications and problems in intramedullary nailing of childrens' fractures.
Eur J Trauma; 26(6):287–293.

Schmittenbecher PP (2004)
Analysis of reinterventions in children's fractures—an aspect of quality control.
Eur J Trauma; 30(2):104–109.

Tarr RR, Garfinkel AI, Sarmiento A
(1984) The effects of angular and rotational deformities of both bones of the forearm. An in-vitro study.
J Bone Joint Surg Am; 66(1):65–70.

Weinberg AM, Kasten P, Castellani C, et al (2001)
Which axial deviation results in limitations of pro- and supination following diaphyseal lower arm fractures in childhood?
Eur J Trauma; 27(6):309–316.

4 Forearm

4.2 Monteggia lesion (22-D/6.1)

1 Case description

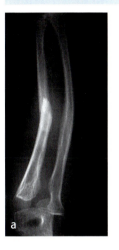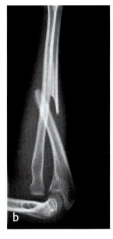

A 12-year-old boy fell at the playground, striking his right forearm against a bar (also known as nightstick fracture in North America). On presentation to the emergency room, he clinically had pain with rotation of the forearm and a visible angular deformity involving the ulnar aspect. The x-rays taken on admission showed a Bado type I Monteggia lesion (Fig 4.2-1).

Fig 4.2-1a–b   Injury x-rays.
a   AP and
b   lateral x-rays showing the characteristic elements of a Bado type I Monteggia lesion.

2 Surgical approach

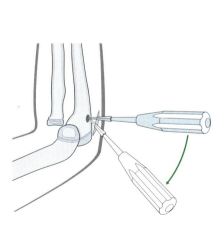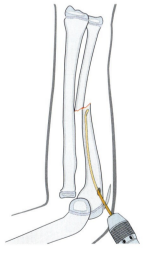

Fig 4.2-2   The tip of the awl is first placed 90° to the lateral cortex and then directed oblique to 45° as it is used to drill the entrance site.

Fig 4.2-3   Antegrade insertion of the nail from the lateral entrance site in the olecranon.

Antegrade approach
To prevent the occurrence of late ulnar angulation and persisting radial head displacement, the ulnar fracture is stabilized by an antegrade approach.

Skin incision
A 2 cm incision is made over the lateral or radial aspect of the olecranon metaphysis starting 2–3 cm distal to the apophysis. Incise directly to the bone.

Entrance site
Once the bone is exposed, a small awl is placed 90° to the lateral cortex (Fig 4.2-2). As the awl is drilled into the medullary canal, it is gradually tilted in an oblique direction.

Nail insertion
A 2–2.5 mm nail is introduced into the entrance site and advanced distally to the fracture (Fig 4.2-3).

4 Forearm

3 Reduction and fixation

Fracture reduction
Once the tip of the nail has reached the fracture site, it is rotated so that it is pointing directly toward the center of the medullary canal of the opposing distal fragment. The fracture fragments are aligned by applying manual pressure with the fingers on the skin directly over the fragments. Additional manipulation of the proximal fragment may be achieved using the nail as a handle (Fig 4.2-4).

Distal advancement
Once the fracture has been aligned, the nail is then manually advanced slowly into the distal fragment. As the nail is fed into the distal fragment, it should correct the deformity of the ulna.

Radial head reduction
Reduction of the ulnar shaft should spontaneously reduce the radial head. The stability and congruency of the radial head reduction are confirmed by rotating the forearm.

Final seating
The nail is cut to place the tip deep in the subcutaneous tissue. The wound is closed with one or two single sutures. To maintain the spread of the interosseous membrane, the tip should be directed toward the radius (Fig 4.2-5).

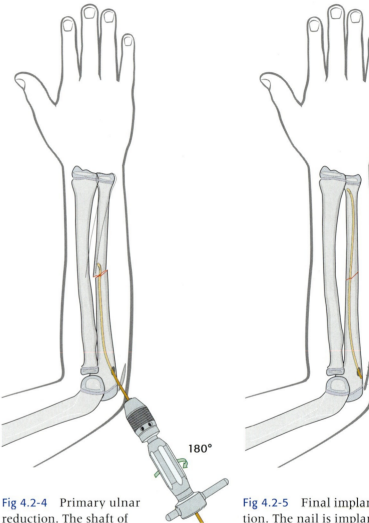

Fig 4.2-4 Primary ulnar reduction. The shaft of the ulna can be reduced with direct pressure on the skin and/or by using the nail as a handle.

Fig 4.2-5 Final implantation. The nail is implanted with the tip directed toward the reduced radius.

4.2 Monteggia lesions (22-D/6.1)

4 Postoperative care and rehabilitation

Early return of function
Since no external immobilization is necessary, free movement can commence when tolerated by the patient. If the postoperative x-rays (Fig 4.2-6) demonstrate satisfactory alignment, the patient can be discharged. If the x-rays at 4 weeks demonstrate adequate consolidation of the ulnar fracture (Fig 4.2-7), sports activities are permitted.

Nail removal
The nail is removed 3–4 months after the injury, providing the x-rays demonstrate complete consolidation (Fig 4.2-8). Once full functional recovery of the forearm has been achieved, further x-rays are no longer necessary.

Role of physiotherapy
Physiotherapy can be helpful if motion continues to be restricted for more than 6 months.

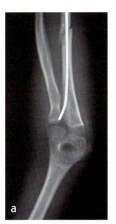 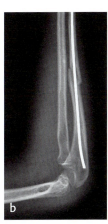 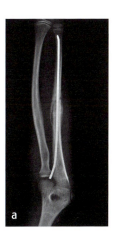 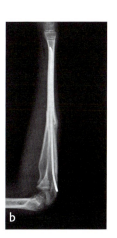 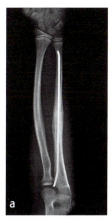 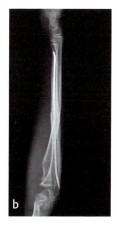

Fig 4.2-6a–b Immediate AP and lateral postoperative x-rays. The radial head dislocation is reduced.

Fig 4.2-7a–b AP and lateral x-rays taken at 4 weeks show early callus and maintenance of the reductions.

Fig 4.2-8a–b AP and lateral x-rays at 4 months demonstrate full healing and considerable consolidation of the ulnar fracture along with maintenance of the radial head reduction. The nail can now be removed.

5 Pitfalls −

Approach
Antegrade nailing of the more proximal fractures of the ulna may lead to an unsatisfactory reduction.

Reduction and fixation
Fig 4.2-9a–d   Persistent displacement of the radial head can lead to a poor outcome. The major cause is usually a residual deformity of the ulna. On rare occasions the radial head does not reduce spontaneously even though the ulna is well aligned (c).

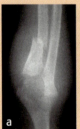
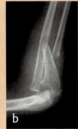
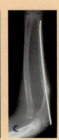
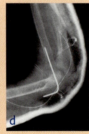

Postoperative care and rehabilitation
Early or aggressive physiotherapy carries a high risk of producing heterotopic ossification around the elbow.

6 Pearls +

Approach
A distal entrance site is preferable in those Monteggia lesions in which the ulnar fracture is proximal.

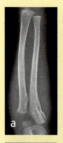
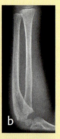

Fig 4.2-10a–b   Example of a Bado type III Monteggia lesion with a very proximal ulnar fracture.

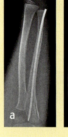
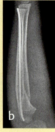

Fig 4.2-11a–b   For these proximal ulnar fractures, retrograde nailing is preferable. The x-rays show reduction of the ulnar fracture and the radial head following retrograde nailing.

Reduction and fixation
- Control the correct position of the radial head intensively using image intensifier during rotation of the forearm and flexion/extension of the elbow.
- If the radius is not spontaneously reduced, try direct reduction by external pressure on the proximal radius.
- If reduction is not reliable, pull out the nail and bend it to effect a more effective and powerful countermovement against the initial ulnar malalignment.
- If bowing of the ulna without any visible fracture is the cause of ongoing radial displacement, use a strong, well prebent ulnar nail. The tension within the nail reduce the plastic deformation of the ulna during the following days.

Postoperative care and rehabilitation
Physiotherapy should be avoided for the first 6 months after the inury.

4.3 Forearm shaft fractures, transverse (12-D/4.1)

1 Case description

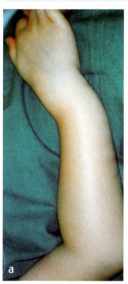
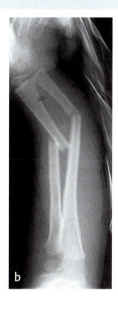
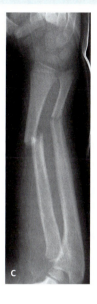

8-year-old boy fell from a tree and presented clinically with an angulated right forearm. The x-rays demonstrated displaced and shortened transverse fractures of the radial and ulnar shafts at nearly the same level (Fig 4.3-1)

Fig 4.3-1a–c
a   Clinical appearance. On presentation, there was an obvious apex-dorsal angulation in the right forearm.
b–c AP and lateral x-rays show complete fractures of the distal shafts of both the radius and ulna with shortening and angulation.

2 Surgical approach

Separate sites
Surgical stabilization of the radial and ulnar shafts requires separate standard insertion sites, one at each end of the forearm. The radial site is distal and the ulnar site is proximal.

Distal dorsal radial nail insertion
A 2–3 cm transverse or longitudinal incision is made over the palpable dorsal tubercle of the radius (Fig 4.3-2). Next, the subcutaneous tissue is spread and the fascia is incised to expose the tubercle. After retracting the incision, the awl is placed directly on the tubercle adjacent to the third compartment containing the extensor tendons. Care is taken to avoid injury to the tendons. The awl is directed anteromedially as it is drilled to perforate the posterior cortex (Fig 4.3-3). At this point it is important to be careful not to perforate the opposite cortex. The nail is introduced and advanced proximally to the fracture site (Fig 4.3-4).

4 Forearm

2 Surgical approach (cont)

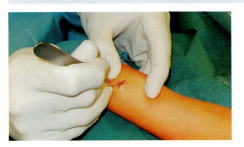

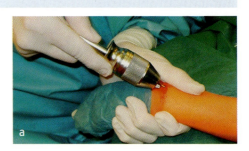

Fig 4.3-2 Radial incision. Small transverse skin incision made over the posterior aspect of the dorsal tubercle of the radius (alternatively longitudinal incision).

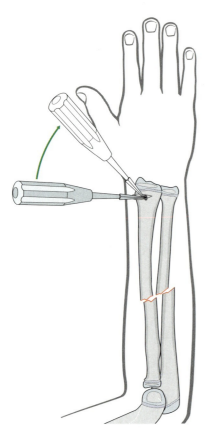

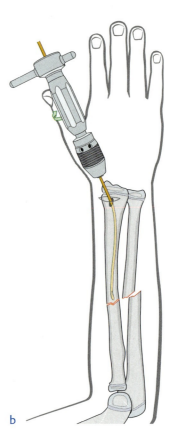

Fig 4.3-3 The radial entrance site is made with the awl first placed perpendicular to the posterior cortex of the tubercle and then directed 45° to enter the medullary canal.

Fig 4.3-4a–b
a Radial nail insertion. The radial nail is inserted into the entrance site and advanced using the T-handled hand chuck.
b Radial nail advancement. Following its insertion, the radial nail is advanced to just short of the fracture site.

4.3 Forearm shaft fractures, transverse (12-D/4.1)

2 Surgical approach (cont)

Proximal ulnar insertion

The skin is incised 1.5–2 cm transversely over the proximal lateral aspect of the olecranon, 3 cm distal to the apophysis. The lateral cortex of the olecranon is perforated with the awl directed obliquely in a distal direction (Fig 4.3-5a). The nail is inserted and advanced distally to the fracture site (Fig 4.3-5b).

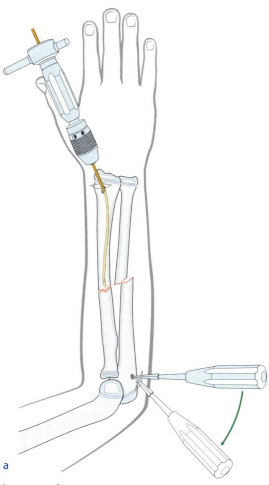

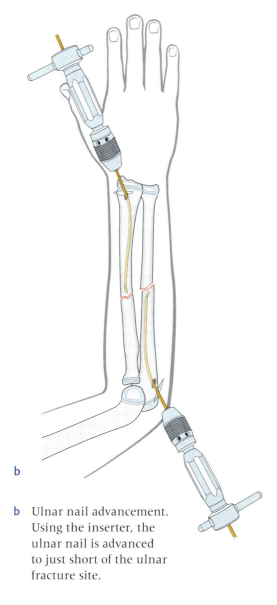

Fig 4.3-5a–b

a   Ulnar entrance site.
    The ulnar site is created on the lateral surface of the olecranon by drilling with the awl first perpendicular to the cortex and then gradually angulating it to enter the medullary canal.

b   Ulnar nail advancement.
    Using the inserter, the ulnar nail is advanced to just short of the ulnar fracture site.

3 Reduction and fixation

3.1 Standard technique—radius

Single reduction
Because it is often the more difficult step, the radius should be reduced first. Attempt to bring the fracture planes in contact indirectly by percutaneously manipulating the proximal fragment. Rotate the radial nail carefully to line up the tip perfectly to the medullary canal of the proximal fragment and then advance the tip into the proximal fragment (Fig 4.3-6). Once passage of the nail into the canal has been verified, the nail is advanced proximally to the level of the radial tuberosity. The tip should be directed toward the ulna (Fig 4.3-7).

Open reduction
Failure to introduce the nail into the proximal fragment requires an open reduction. To do so, make a short incision at the level of the fracture to remove the obstructing soft tissue. Under direct vision, reduce the fracture with small clamps and then advance the tip of the nail into the proximal fragment (Fig 4.3-8).

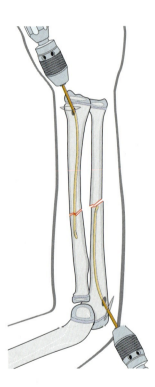

Fig 4.3-6 Radial reduction.
Once reduction of the radius has been achieved, the radial nail is advanced into the proximal fragment.

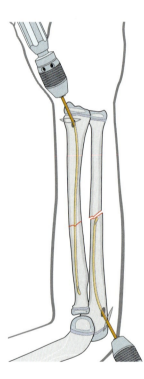

Fig 4.3-7 Radial positioning.
This nail is advanced proximally to the level of the radial tuberosity. The tip is directed toward the ulna.

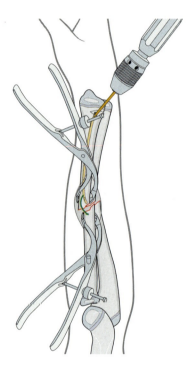

Fig 4.3-8 Open reduction.
Failure to achieve a closed reduction may require exposure of the fracture site through a small incision to visualize passage of the tip into the proximal fragment.

4.3 Forearm shaft fractures, transverse (12-D/4.1)

3 Reduction and fixation (cont)

3.2 Standard technique—ulna

Single reduction
Following reduction of the radius, the ulna usually reduces spontaneously. The ulnar nail is advanced distally to the distal ulnar metaphysis. It is then secured in the strong cancellous metaphyseal bone with the tip rotated toward the radius to produce maximal spreading of the interosseous membrane (Fig 4.3-9). On rare occasions the ulna may need an open reduction in the same manner as described for the radius.

Simultaneous reduction
If reduction of the radius and/or ulna is difficult, it may be helpful initially to only advance the radial nail as far as the fracture site. Then, proceed with the insertion of the ulnar nail. Now, the reduction can often be accomplished more easily because both nails can be manipulated simultaneously.

3.3 Final position of both nails

The nails are cut and their ends placed deep in the subcutaneous tissue. The incisions are then closed with single sutures (Fig 4.3-10). The end of the radial nail must be placed sufficiently outside the tendon compartment to prevent constant friction and tendon rupture.

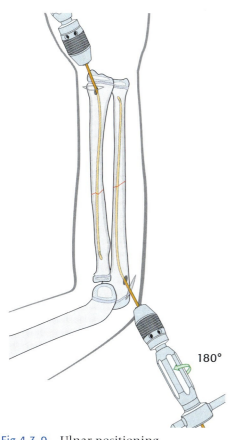

Fig 4.3-9 Ulnar positioning.
The ulnar nail is advanced distally to seat the tip in the metaphysis. The tip should be directed toward the radius.

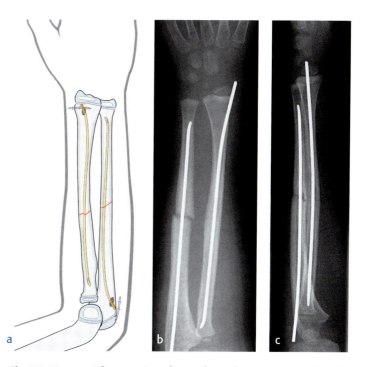

Fig 4.3-10a–c After cutting the nails to the proper length, the ends are buried under the subcutaneous tissues. Notice the spreading effect on the interosseous membrane produced by central pointing of the tips (see Fig 4.1-3).

4   Forearm

3   Reduction and fixation   (cont)

3.4 Alternative techniques—radius

Many surgeons prefer to insert the radial nail by a lateral approach on the distal radius. The incision here needs to be a little longer in order to identify and protect the superficial radial nerve. The awl must carefully be placed directly on the lateral cortex (Fig 4.3-11).

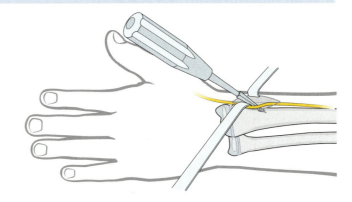

Fig 4.3-11   Lateral radial incision. Alternatively, the distal radial entrance site can be placed in the lateral cortex. It is important to be sure that the incision is long enough to visualize and retract the superficial radial nerve.

3.5 Alternative techniques—ulna

Insertion of the ulnar nail in its distal metaphysis is favored by many surgeons. An incision is placed over the distal medial ulnar metaphysis. The medullary canal is opened with the awl and the nail is introduced and advanced in retrograde technique (see chapter 4.6, Fig 4.6-2 to Fig 4.6-5). Manipulation of both bones from the same end may be helpful in reducing difficult fracture patterns.

Fig 4.3-12a–d
a–b   Both nails are introduced retrograde through the entrance site in the distal metaphysis. Postoperative x-rays demonstrate ESIN stabilization with correct axial alignment.
c–d   Detailed view of the distal ulnar entry point on image intensifier.

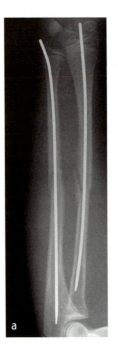
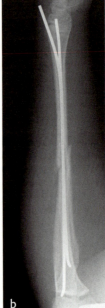
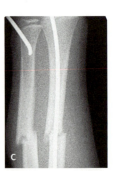
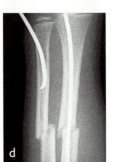

4.3 Forearm shaft fractures, transverse (12-D/4.1)

4 Postoperative care and rehabilitation

Early motion allowed

The postoperative x-rays demonstrate a satisfactory final alignment (Fig 4.3-13). Because no postoperative immobilization is required, active motion can commence as tolerated (Fig 4.3-14). X-rays 4 weeks later demonstrate sufficient callus formation (Fig 4.3-15) to permit participation in sports. At 3 months postinjury, the x-rays demonstrate sufficient consolidation and remodeling to schedule nail removal (Fig 4.3-16). In most cases, there is full functional recovery (Fig 4.3-17).

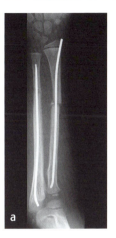
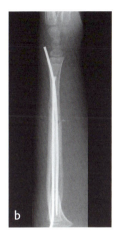
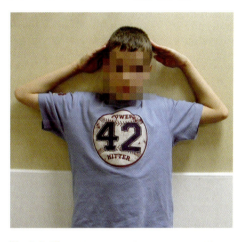
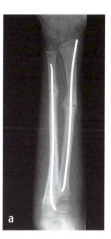
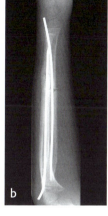

Fig 4.3-13a–b Postoperative x-rays taken immediately after ESIN stabilization.

Fig 4.3-14 Almost full recovery of elbow motion 5 days after ESIN stabilization of the radial and ulnar shafts.

Fig 4.3-15a–b X-rays at 4 weeks show early callus formation.

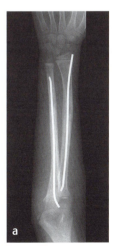
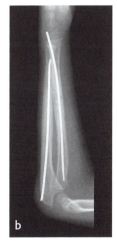
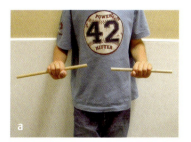
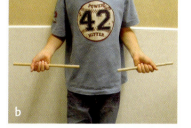

Fig 4.3-16a–b AP and lateral x-rays taken 3 months later prior to removal of the nails. Almost complete remodeling of the fracture site.

Fig 4.3-17a–b This young boy has recovered full supination (a) and pronation (b).

5 Pitfalls −

Approach

Avoid performing the posterior radial approach totally percutaneously (without a surgical incision) as this may injure one of the extensor tendons.

Take great care not to perforate the opposite cortex when inserting the awl. Perforating the cortex will produce an abnormal passageway that will guide the nail into the vital anterior or medial soft tissues which can then become injured.

Always be sure that the cut end of the nail lies outside the tendon compartment. A secondary tendon injury could arise from constant rubbing against the sharp end of nail (Fig 4.3-18).

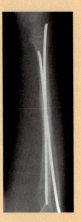

Fig 4.3-18 Tendon rupture. In this case the extensor pollicis longus tendon was ruptured by rubbing against the sharp edge of the short radial nail. This happens if the direction of the nail is very flat and the nail is cut very short.

Avoid implantation of the ulnar nail directly through the olecranon apophysis. The cut end of the nail will lie very superficially which would allow it to perforate the skin easily.

Antegrade radial nailing with its proximal insertion carries a high risk of injury to the deep branch of the radial nerve. This approach and technique should never be used!

6 Pearls +

Approach

Incising the skin sufficiently and retracting it with small hooks to allow placement of the awl under direct view will prevent this complication.

Accentuation of the curve of the nail tips will facilitate their gliding off the inner surface of the opposite metaphyseal cortex. This will guide the tip into the medullary canal.

The posteriorly implanted radial nail should be long enough to lie outside the extensor tendon compartment in the subcutaneous tissue.

Insert the ulnar nail through the lateral cortex of the olecranon a few centimeters distal to the tip.

5 Pitfalls – (cont)

Reduction and fixation

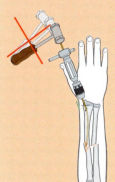

Too aggressive manipulation of the nail at the fracture site can blow out a small fragment, making it difficult to align the fracture.

Fig 4.3-19 Fracture blow-out. Forcing a nail through the narrow diaphyseal canal using a hammer can produce a blow-out fragment.

Rehabilitation

There is a high risk of refracture if premature removal of the nails is performed before there is definitive consolidation of the fracture.

6 Pearls + (cont)

Reduction and fixation

In those areas where the medullary canal is very narrow, advance the nail only by hand. Do not use a hammer. Do not try to advance the nail by force if there is a lot of resistance. The nail can be advanced by gradually rotating its tip.

Rehabilitation

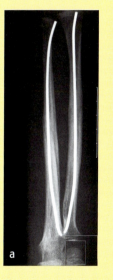 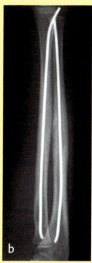

Fig 4.3-20a–b Removal should not be performed until there is x-ray evidence of solid union and remodeling at the fracture site.

5 Pitfalls − (cont)

Rehabilitation (cont)

If significant restriction of pronation or supination continues for more than 3 months after nail removal, physiotherapy should be initiated with close supervision until full functional recovery has been achieved.

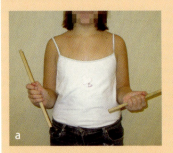
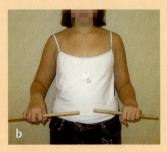
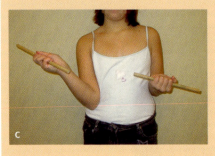

Fig 4.3-21a–c Patient demonstrating limitation of supination (a) and pronation (b). Notice the compensation by the shoulder (c).

6 Pearls + (cont)

4.4 Radial and ulnar shaft fractures, displaced radius with butterfly fragment, ulna simple (12-D/5.2)

1 Case description

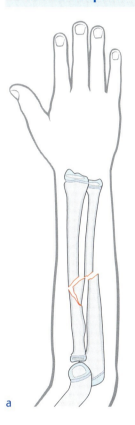
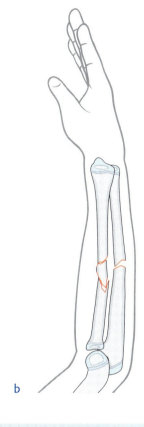

A 14-year-old male involved in a scooter accident presented with a visible angular deformity of his right forearm. His x-rays demonstrated displaced radial and ulnar shaft fractures with a large butterfly fragment of the radius and a transverse fracture of the ulna (Fig 4.4-1).

Fig 4.4-1a–b Schematic representation demonstrating the acute fracture pattern with the presence of a large butterfly fragment in the midshaft of the radius.
a AP view.
b Lateral view.

Prerequisites for ESIN stabilization
ESIN can be performed with these fracture patterns, providing the main fragments of the radius maintain both adequate contact and length, and the alignment can be stabilized.

a
b

2 Surgical approach

Stabilization of the radius
Start with the radius, utilizing the same approach as demonstrated in the case presented in chapter 4.3 Forearm shaft fractures, transverse (see Figs 4.3-3 to 4.3-7). Stabilization of the radius should be completed prior to stabilization of the ulna to be sure that a satisfactory reduction can be achieved.

Stabilization of the ulna
Ulna stabilization. After the radial nail is well secured in the region of the radial neck, the ulna is stabilized as outlined in the aforementioned case in chapter 4.3 Forearm shaft fractures, transverse (see Figs 4.3-5 to 4.3-9). As an alternate technique, distal retrograde implantation of the ulnar nail can be satisfactorily accomplished as described in Figs 4.3-3 to 4.3-5.

4 Forearm

3 Reduction and fixation

Radial stabilization
Reaching the fracture region, rotate the tip of the nail so that a displacement of the wedge is avoided. If the tip of the nail faces the tip of the wedge, the nail may glide along the base side of the wedge.

Direct manipulation
Externally reduce the main fragments by directly manipulating the distal fragment with the implanted nail to bring the planes of the fracture fragments into direct apposition (Fig 4.4-2).

Proximal insertion
Insert the nail into the proximal medullary canal and advance it proximally to the area of the radial neck (Fig 4.4-3). At this point evaluate the alignment and stability of the reduction of the radius. The wedge can remain in its original position in the surrounding soft tissue, as long as it does not impinge on the interosseous membrane.

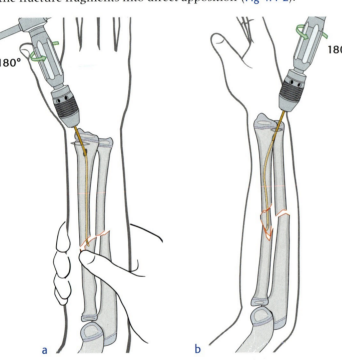

Fig 4.4-2a–b
a The fragments are manually reduced and held as the tip of the nail is introduced into the fracture site. At this point the nail should glide on the base of the butterfly to facilitate entrance into the fragment.
b Once the fragment has been entered, the nail is rotated to place the blunt surface against the intact cortex of the fragment so as to avoid displacing it.

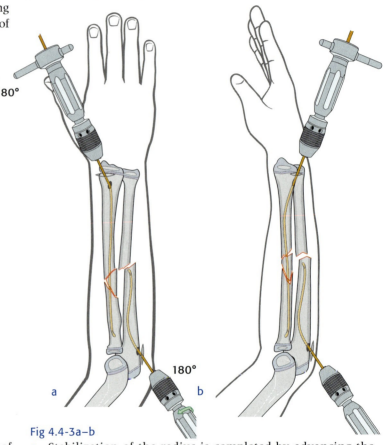

Fig 4.4-3a–b
a Stabilization of the radius is completed by advancing the nail tip proximally to the level of the radial neck.
b Ulnar stabilization. The nail is then inserted into the proximal ulna and passed antegrade to the fracture site.

4.4 Radial and ulnar shaft fractures, displaced radius with butterfly fragment, ulna simple (12-D/5.2)

3 Reduction and fixation (cont)

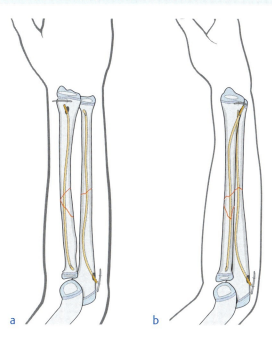

Final nail placement
Once the radius is aligned, the ulnar nail can easily be advanced antegrade into the distal fragment (Fig 4.4-3). In the final position, the tips of both nails are directed toward the interosseous membrane. The blunt ends of the nails are cut at the correct length and are buried in the subcutaneous tissue. The skin is closed with single sutures (Fig 4.4-4).

If there is insufficient stability to allow unprotected motion, ESIN should be abandoned and the fracture stabilized by other means such as an external fixator. Therefore, stability has to be proven before the end of anesthesia.

Fig 4.4-4a–b After having reduced the fracture and advanced the ulnar nail distally to the distal metaphysis, the blunt ends of both nails are cut to leave only a small portion outside the cortex. Notice that the tips of both nails are directed toward the interosseous membrane to enhance the stability.

4 Postoperative care and rehabilitation

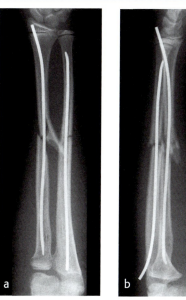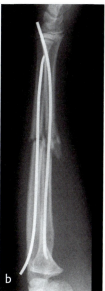

Mobility encouraged
Postoperative cast immobilization is not necessary. Control x-rays should be taken prior to discharge (Fig 4.4-5).

Fig 4.4-5a–b Postoperative x-rays showing the anterior wedge without interposition into the interosseous membrane.
a AP view.
b Lateral view.

4 Postoperative care and rehabilitation (cont)

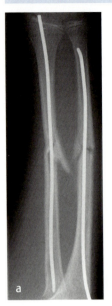
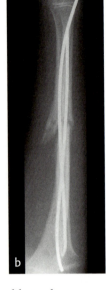
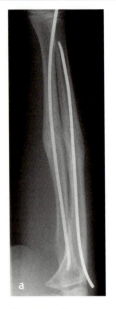
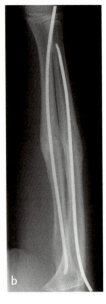

Fig 4.4-6a–b AP and lateral x-rays at 4 weeks.

Fig 4.4-7a-b AP and lateral x-rays at 4 months.

Fragment incorporation
X-rays obtained 4 weeks later should confirm good callus formation with incorporation of the wedge (Fig 4.4-6). Forearm rotation is evaluated clinically. It is expected that there may still be some limitation at this time. By 4 months postoperative, the wedge should be completely reintegrated and remodeled into the main fragment (Fig 4.4-7).

Final follow-up
Once the fracture is fully consolidated, the nails can be safely removed. The patient should be followed clinically until a satisfactory functional outcome has been achieved.

5 Pitfalls –

Reduction and fixation
The radial nail is unable to straighten and/or stabilize the radius into a satisfactory anatomical alignment because there is insufficient contact of the main fragments. This allows the contacting fragment tips to slide along each other.

Intraoperatively, the wedge is displaced significantly between radius and ulna to compromise forearm rotation.

Rehabilitation
Too early mobilization with sports or loading activities results in a secondary displacement.

6 Pearls +

Reduction and fixation
The axial reconstruction of the radius should be evaluated by rotating the forearm under real-time image intensification. If stability has not been achieved, the stabilization technique should be converted to another method, such as an external fixator.

Surgically explore the fracture site and bring the wedge into better contact to the radius.

If the position of the wedge alone was the problem and the surgical stabilization is acceptable, the original technique need not be changed.

Rehabilitation
In multifragmentary fractures, postoperative rehabilitation may have to be restricted to prevent redisplacement.

4.5 Radial and ulnar shaft fractures, malunion following conservative treatment (22-D/4.1)

1 Case description

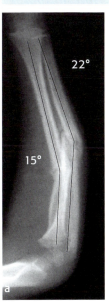
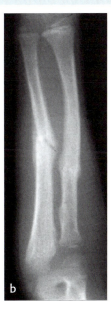

A 6-year-old boy sustained displaced fractures of the left radial and ulnar shafts. He had previously undergone conservative treatment at another medical facility with a long-arm cast for 4 weeks. X-rays on completion of his treatment revealed united fractures with significant malalignment (Fig 4.5-1). Clinically, there was severe restriction of supination and pronation.

ESIN gives the opportunity to correct the malalignment indirectly without osteotomy as long as the medullary canal is visible.

Fig 4.5-1a–b X-rays taken after cast removal showed 15° of angulation of the radial shaft and 22° of the ulnar shaft. The fracture sites were united with abundant callus.
a   Lateral view.
b   AP view.

2 Surgical approach

Both nails can be implanted as described previously in the case presented in chapter 4.3 Forearm shaft fracture, transverse (see Figs 4.3-3 to 4.3-10). If the reduction of the radius (or of the ulna) is not sufficient to allow insertion of the nail into the intramedullary canal of the proximal fragment, then an open reduction needs to be performed. Often in previous healed fractures, the medullary canal is obstructed by callus which may require an open approach and drilling to facilitate passage of the nail tip.

3 Reduction and fixation

Surgical exposure

The nail is inserted into the distal radius via a dorsal entrance site and advanced to just short of the fracture site. The fracture site of the radius is then exposed surgically through a 3–4 cm skin incision. Next, the fascia is opened and the tissue planes between the forearm extensor and thumb flexor muscles are separated carefully to expose the fracture fragments (Fig 4.5-2). The interposed muscle tissue is removed to clear and free the fragments. Once the soft-tissue impediments have been removed, the fracture can easily be reduced with a small hook or clamp. At this point the nail can easily be introduced into the medullary canal and advanced proximally to the radial neck. The fracture is then managed to complete the osteosynthesis as in the case presented in chapter 4.3 Forearm shaft fractures, transverse (see Figs 4.3-8 to 4.3-10).

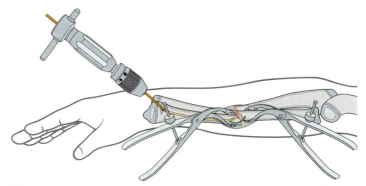

Fig 4.5-2 Open reduction. Following exposure of the fracture site through a 3–4 cm skin incision, the fracture is reduced with small reduction forceps to facilitate direct introduction of the nail into the medullary canal of the proximal fragment.

4 Postoperative care and rehabilitation

The postoperative management is the same as previously described with routine radial and ulnar shaft fractures. Postoperative and follow-up course is shown in Figs 4.5-3 to 4.5-5. The x-rays at 3 months usually demonstrate complete healing and remodeling (Fig 4.5-5) sufficient to allow nail removal. If, however, there is insufficient callus formation, removal of the nails should be postponed.

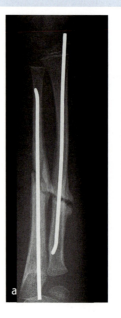 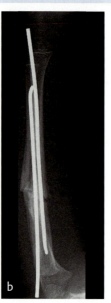

Fig 4.5-3a–b X-rays taken immediately postoperatively show correction of the angular deformity.

4.5 Radial and ulnar shaft fractures, malunion following conservative treatment (22-D/4.1)

4 Postoperative care and rehabilitation (cont)

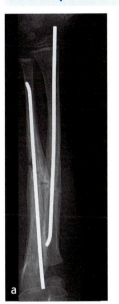
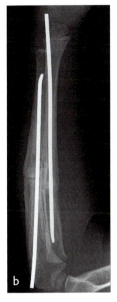

Fig 4.5-4a–b X-rays taken at 4 weeks show early obliteration of the fracture line and early callus.

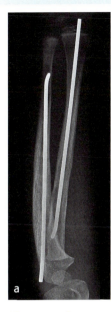
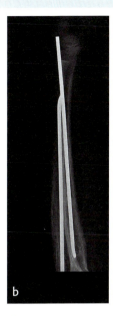

Fig 4.5-5a–b X-rays taken at 3 months: there was sufficient obliteration of the fracture line and remodeling of the callus to allow nail removal.

5 Pitfalls –

Reduction and fixation
Using an incision at the fracture site that is too short for the open reduction.

Making too many attempts to obtain a reduction by closed manipulation.

6 Pearls +

Reduction and fixation
Because of the need to perform vigorous retraction with a small incision, there may be more soft-tissue trauma with a short incision than with an adequate skin incision which easily provides sufficient visualization of the tissues involved.

The treating surgeon needs to understand that there is a risk of soft-tissue injury plus radiation exposure by repeated unsuccessful manipulations to achieve a closed reduction. These risks need to be weighed against the relatively controlled soft-tissue trauma of an open reduction. The decision to perform an open procedure is determined by the surgeon's judgment and skill.

4 Forearm

4.6 Radial and ulnar shaft refracture after conservative treatment (22-D/4.1)

1 Case description

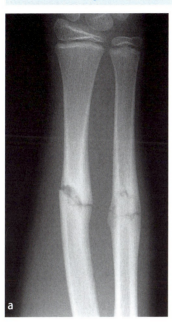
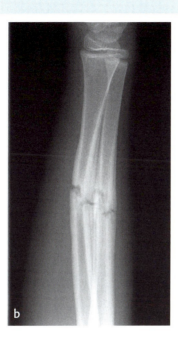

9-year-old boy who fell over 2 months after cast removal. Refractures of the radial and ulnar shafts of his previously conservatively treated fractures.

Fig 4.6-1a–b AP and lateral x-rays showing refractures of the shafts of the radius and ulna.

2 Surgical approach

Drilling of canal

Refractures in the radial and ulnar shafts can be stabilized with ESIN using the same technique as that used for the malaligned fractures. Closed reduction of these refractures may be difficult because the ends of the fragments may be covered with callus. If a good intramedullary canal is not identifiable on the x-ray, ESIN may not be possible by closed methods. The medullary canals have to be cleared by drilling the exposed fracture surfaces.

4 Forearm

2 Surgical approach (cont)

Retrograde approach

Again, if implantation of the nails of one or both of the forearm bones is expected to be difficult, it may be best to approach both the radius and ulna "in the same direction". This would require a retrograde approach for both fractures. The radius is first stabilized via the standard retrograde approach. To stabilize the ulna via the retrograde approach, a 2–3 cm incision over the distal ulna is made starting 3 cm proximal to the palpable ulnar styloid (Fig 4.6-2). The dissection is carefully continued directly to the bone. The awl is placed 90° to the ulna and then drilled obliquely to produce the entrance site, taking care to prevent perforation of the opposite cortex (Fig 4.6-3).

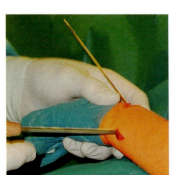

Fig 4.6-2 Distal skin incisions. The radius has been stabilized by the standard retrograde approach with a dorsal distal entrance site. The distal ulnar entrance site is made with the awl using an incision 3 cm proximal to the prominence of the ulnar styloid.

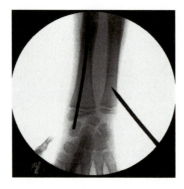

Fig 4.6-3 Ulnar entrance site. In creating the entrance site in the distal ulna, the awl is directed obliquely proximal to facilitate the initial passage of the nail and avoid penetration of the opposite cortex.

3 Reduction and fixation

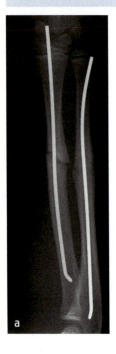
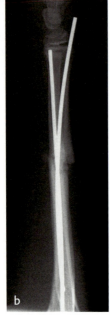

The nail is inserted and carefully advanced proximally in retrograde technique to the level of the olecranon to secure rigid stabilization (Fig 4.6-4).

This insertion should be performed with caution because of the small medullary canal. If the stabilization and position of the nails is satisfactory, the incisions over the distal entrance sites are closed with simple sutures (Fig 4.6-5).

Fig 4.6-4a–b AP and lateral x-rays taken immediately postoperative. The tip of the nail on the radius lies at the level of the radial tuberosity and that of the ulnar nail lies at the level of the coronoid process. Note that the tips of the nails are directed toward each other which enhances separation of the interosseous membrane.

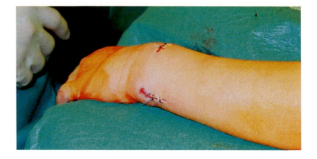

Fig 4.6-5 Skin closure. The incisions over the entrance site are closed with simple sutures.

4.6 Radial and ulnar shaft refracture after conservative treatment (22-D/4.1)

4 Postoperative care and rehabilitation

If adequate stabilization is achieved, the patient is allowed to begin motion of the forearm as relief of the operative pain permits. X-rays are taken at 4 weeks (Fig 4.6-6) and 3 months (Fig 4.6-7). Nail removal can be accomplished when full healing and remodeling of the fracture has been achieved.

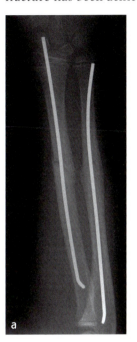
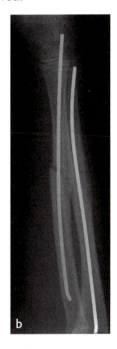
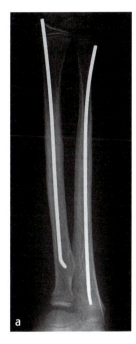
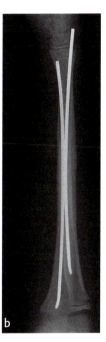

Fig 4.6-6a–b AP and lateral x-rays taken 4 weeks postoperatively demonstrate early callus and maintenance of the original reduction.

Fig 4.6-7a–b 3-month follow-up x-rays demonstrate complete healing and remodeling of the fracture sites. The nails can be safely removed at this time.

4 Forearm

4.7 Distal radial and ulnar diaphyseal-metaphyseal fractures, displaced (22-D/4.1)

1 Case description

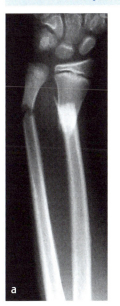
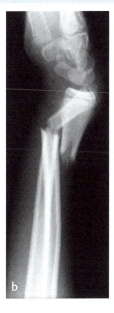

A 13-year-old male who had sustained severe head trauma as a result of an accident between a motor vehicle and a bicycle; he also had a displaced fracture of the distal radius at the transition zone between the metaphysis and diaphysis (Fig 4.7-1). The fracture site was too proximal from the distal end to use typical K-wire fixation.

Fig 4.7-1a–b AP and lateral x-rays demonstrating transverse fractures of both the radius and ulna at the diaphyseal–metaphyseal junction.

2 Surgical approach

Radial insertion
The skin is transversely incised posteriorly over the palpable radial tubercle as described in the case presented in Fig 4.3-3 in chapter 4.3 Forearm shaft fracture, transverse. The tendon compartments are opened to expose the bone. The awl is placed posteromedial to the tubercle and drilled almost perpendicular to the cortex to enter the medullary canal directly. Next, the nail is inserted and guided in such a way that it contacts the opposite cortex before it reaches the fracture site (Fig 4.7-2). To facilitate nail advancement in this manner, the tip may need to have a greater bend. Because of the degree of curvature required, advancement of the nail may be difficult. The nail needs to be advanced slowly and carefully. It is advisable to avoid using a hammer as it may blow out a fragment.

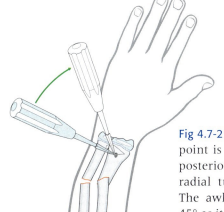

Fig 4.7-2 The radial entry point is created distally in the posterior cortex of the palpable radial tubercle using an awl. The awl is gradually directed 45° as it drills through the cortex (curved arrow).

4 Forearm

2 Surgical approach (cont)

Ulnar insertion
In the ulna, the skin is incised proximally on the lateral aspect of the olecranon 3 cm distal to the tip of the apophysis. The awl is used to create the entrance site by first inserting it perpendicularly to the lateral cortex and then directing it distally as it is drilled through the cortex (Fig 4.7-3). The nail is inserted and advanced to the fracture site in a antegrade manner as described in the case presented in Figs 4.3-5 to 4.3-7 in chapter 4.3 Forearm shaft fractures, transverse.

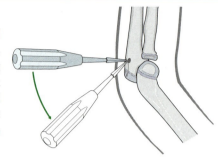

Fig 4.7-3 The entrance site is made in the lateral cortex of the proximal ulna. The awl is gradually directed 45° as it is drilled through the cortex (curved arrow).

3 Reduction and fixation

Radial reduction
First, the nail is advanced proximally to the fracture site. At the same time the nail in the ulna is advanced distally to its fracture site (Fig 4.7-4). This allows the nails to be utilized, if necessary, as lever arms to facilitate manipulation of the fragments. The radius is indirectly reduced externally by manipulating the longer proximal fragment by hand while simultaneously manipulating the distal fragment with the nail. When sufficient apposition of the fracture surfaces has been achieved, the nail is advanced into the proximal fragment.

Alignment correction
Often the nail will not cause the distal fragment to align accurately. The distal radius tends to drift into a valgus position. To correct this, the surgeon needs to assess the point on the nail which will lie at the fracture site when it is finally implanted. Prior to its final insertion, the nail is significantly prebent in its distal portion at that predicted level which will lie at the fracture site (Fig 4.7-5a). The nail is then advanced to place the prebent portion exactly at the fracture site. Once it is fully inserted, the nail is rotated to place the apex of the bend in the plane of maximum malalignment (Fig 4.7-5b). This should provide a satisfactory linear alignment of the fracture fragments. The nail is cut and the end placed in the subcutaneous tissue followed by closure of the incision.

Ulnar reduction
The distal ulna is easy to stabilize with antegrade nailing. The short distal fragment has a narrow medullary canal which provides good internal stability for the nail. Once both nails are in their final position there should be a satisfactory linear and rotational alignment of the fracture fragments (Fig 4.7-6).

4.7 Distal radial and ulnar diaphyseal-metaphyseal fractures, displaced (22-D/4.1)

3 Reduction and fixation (cont)

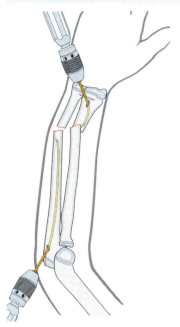
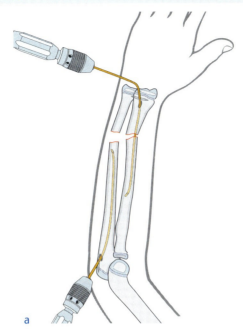
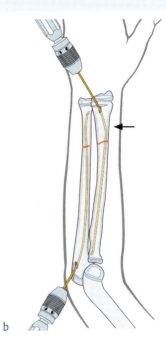

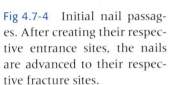

Fig 4.7-4 Initial nail passages. After creating their respective entrance sites, the nails are advanced to their respective fracture sites.

Fig 4.7-5a–b Alignment correction.
a The radial nail is bent distally at the area predetermined to lie at the fracture site. The bend is created so as to resist the tendency of the fracture to drift into valgus malalignment.
b In its final position, the apex of the bend (arrow) has been rotated at the fracture site so that it forces the distal fragment into satisfactory alignment.

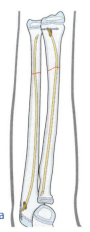
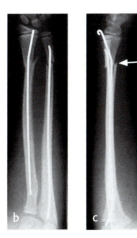

Fig 4.7-6a–c
a   Final position of the inserted nails.
b–c AP and lateral x-rays taken postoperatively demonstrating a satisfactory reduction of the fracture fragments. Note also, the apex of the secondary bend of the radial nail (arrow) is at the fracture site.

105

4 Postoperative care and rehabilitation

The postoperative management (Fig 4.7-7) is the same as for the other forearm shaft fractures treated by the ESIN technique. Since an additional cast is not indicated, motion can be initiated as soon as the patient can tolerate it. If the stability of the intramedullary fixation seems to be inadequate to guarantee alignment of the fracture fragments, then the ESIN technique is not appropriate and the fracture should be stabilized by another method such as a small external fixator.

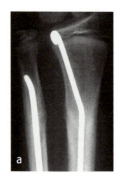 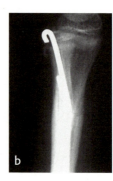

Fig 4.7-7a–b   Final healing prior to nail removal. AP and lateral x-rays. The initial reduction has been maintained and there is good remodeling of the fracture callus.

5 Pitfalls –

Approach

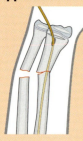

Fig 4.7-8   Too much obliquity in inserting the radial nail causes the nail to pass the fracture site before it contacts the opposite cortex of the distal fragment. This does not allow sufficient stability to maintain the alignment of the fracture fragments.

If a hammer is used to advance the nail in the thin metaphyseal segment, there is the danger that it will blow out a fragment.

6 Pearls +

Approach
Introduce the radial nail almost perpendicular to the cortex. If the lateral insertion site produces too oblique an angle, change to a posterior insertion site. The same is true if the posterior site is too oblique.

Never use the hammer at these points of insertion. If a fragment is blown out, there is almost no chance of obtaining a stable reduction with this technique. Stabilization of the fracture may require converting to the use of an external fixator.

4.7 Distal radial and ulnar diaphyseal-metaphyseal fractures, displaced (22-D/4.1)

5 Pitfalls – (cont)

Approach   (cont)

In those cases where it is not possible to obtain a stable reduction with retrograde fixation, it must be remembered that antegrade radial nailing risks injury to the deep branch of the radial nerve (Fig 4.7-9).

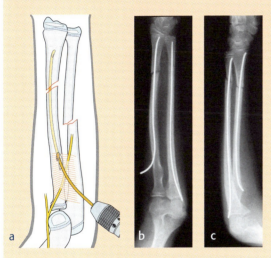

Fig 4.7-9a–c   Avoid proximal radial insertion.
a   This line drawing demonstrates the proximity of the radial nerve to a proximal insertion site in the radius.
b–c   AP and lateral x-rays of a patient who had the radial nail inserted proximally. The fractures have healed but there was a profound radial nerve paralysis.

Reduction and fixation

Failure to fully evaluate the final anatomical alignment at the fracture site may result in an unsatisfactory alignment of the distal fragment.

6 Pearls + (cont)

Approach   (cont)

Antegrade nailing of the radius is a problematic solution for this situation. It is better to use an external fixator (Fig 4.7-10).

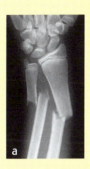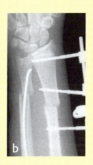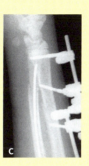

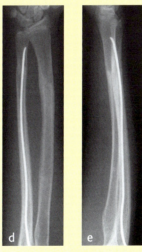

Fig 4.7-10a–e
a   Displaced distal meta-diaphyseal forearm fracture, too close to the physis to use ESIN for the radius, to far from the physis to use K-wires.
b–c   Decision for a fixation of the radius with a small external fixator and ESIN stabilization of the ulna. The postoperative x-ray shows a good alignment.
d–e   After 4 weeks, the external fixator was removed without any anesthesia.

Reduction and fixation

Careful evaluation and control of the nail is always very important in all the stages of managing these metaphyseal-diaphyseal fractures. If needed, the radial nail should be withdrawn and its curvature accentuated. The nail must then be replaced or exchanged.

5 Femur

5.1 **Introduction—femoral fractures** 109
- 1 Indication 109
- 2 Patient preparation and positioning 109
- 3 Surgical principles 111
- 4 Implant removal 111
- 5 Suggested reading 112

5.2 **Proximal femoral fracture, subtrochanteric (32-D/5.1)** 113

5.3 **Femoral shaft fracture, transverse (32-D/4.1)** 119

5.4 **Femoral shaft refracture, oblique (32-D/5.1)** 129

5.5 **Segmental femoral shaft fracture (32-D/5.2) and ipsilateral tibial shaft fracture (42-D/5.1)** 135

5.6 **Distal femoral fracture (33-M/3.1)** 141

5.1 Introduction—femoral fractures

1 Indication

Nonoperative treatment in the younger patient
Because healing is rapid, nonoperative techniques such as hip spica casts with or without preliminary traction are the preferred management in the 1–3 year age group. Another reason that conservative management is recommended in these younger patients is the suspected risk of overgrowth with ESIN. Since very little experience has been gained with ESIN in this very young age group, the extent of possible complications has not been determined.

Surgery—age dependent
The most commonly accepted indication for operative intervention of femoral shaft fractures is for the 3–15 year age group. The decision to utilize the ESIN technique is based upon many factors. These may include the presence of other injuries or health conditions or the size and age of the patient. The experience of the surgeon can also be a factor in the decision making.

Advantages of ESIN
As outlined in chapter 1 Basic principles dealing with the basics principles of ESIN, this technique stabilizes the fracture utilizing a minimally invasive technique. In most cases stability is sufficient to allow early motion and protected weight bearing. This in turn decreases the time needed to achieve a full return to normal function.

2 Patient preparation and positioning

Patient preparation
These patients need to be both hemodynamically and neurologically stable prior to their surgical procedures. In certain situations where the fractures are open or there is neurovascular compromise, the surgical procedure may need to be performed under emergency or urgent conditions.

Medication
The protocol regarding the use of prophylactic antibiotics is based upon the standard of care in the clinic protocol. Likewise, the standard guidelines should also be followed regarding the use of thrombosis prophylaxis in females who are postmenarchal, patients with pelvic trauma, or those patients who are overweight.

Patient positioning
ESIN in patients with femoral fractures is performed with the patient lying supine either on a standard fracture table or suspended in traction on the pediatric orthopedic table depending upon the experience and preference of the treating surgeon. The use of the orthopedic table may greatly facilitate the insertion of the nails in those instances where minimal surgical assistance is available, in children whose fractures are transverse, or in the larger older child.

5 Femur

2 Patient preparation and positioning (cont)

The proper position of the patient on the standard operating table along with the positioning of the intact lower extremity is demonstrated in Fig 5.1-1. The alternative position of the patient in traction on the pediatric orthopedic table is seen in Fig 5.1-2.

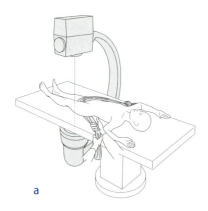
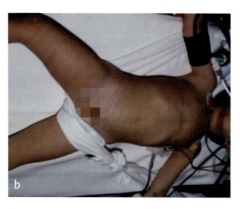
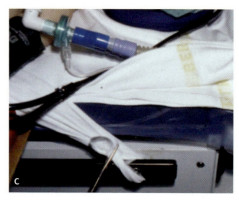

Fig 5.1-1a–c Positioning on a standard table.
a Position of the patient on the standard operating table.

b Clinical photo demonstrating the position of the patient. A folded sheet is placed around the proximal portion of the extremity involved to provide countertraction.

c The sheet is attached to the side of the table with a large surgical clamp.

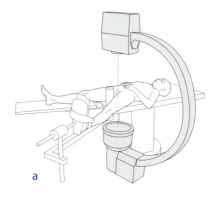
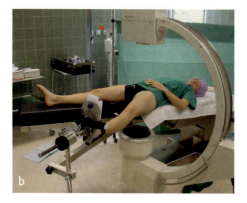

Fig 5.1-2a-b Positioning an a traction table.
a Patient suspended in traction on an orthopedic table. The uninjured lower extremity should be at the same level as the injured extremity unless there is no other way to obtain adequate imaging.
b Clinical photo of a patient on the traction table.

5.1 Introduction—femoral fractures

2 Patient preparation and positioning (cont)

Preparation for the surgical procedure
Prior to performing the surgical technique, certain preoperative preparations are needed regarding the equipment required. Decisions also need to be made regarding the selection of the appropriate nails and the surgical approaches.

The fracture pattern determines the direction of nailing, which, in turn, determines the positioning of the patient and the image intensifier prior to the actual procedure. It will also determine the location of the primary surgical incision. For antegrade nailing the nail is inserted into the subtrochanteric area. For retrograde nailing the nail is inserted into the distal part of the femur.

Equipment
In addition to the standard surgical instruments used to treat any long-bone fracture, the minimal requirements to manage femoral fractures with the ESIN technique include:
- Standard ESIN set.
- Nails:
  2.0–5.0 mm diameter stainless steel or titanium; the selected nails should be 33% (1/3) of the diameter of the intramedullary canal.
- Image intensifier.

3 Surgical principles

In discussing the surgical management of femoral fractures in children, they will be divided into the following subgroups based upon location and type of fracture pattern:

The specific surgical techniques for all subtypes (location and fracture pattern) of femoral fractures in children will be discussed in their respective subchapters to follow:
- 5.2 Subtrochanteric fractures
- 5.3 Transverse and spiral shaft fractures
- 5.4 Refracture following application of an external fixator
- 5.5 Segmental and ipsilateral fractures (polytrauma)

4 Implant removal

Timing of removal
X-rays are taken just prior to nail removal. Depending on age, fracture type and site, and the level of recovery, this period can range from 6–12 months (exeptionally, 4 months may suffice) following surgery.

Extraction techniques
The old incision site is utilized to expose the nail end. After first removing the cap (if plastic caps or end caps were used), locking pliers are used to grasp the end of the nail. The nail is then carefully removed. Sometimes the nail end is positioned too close to the bone to allow the extraction tool to obtain a secure grasp. If this is the case, the nail end is simply bent sufficiently away from the cortex to permit safe extraction.

If the nail appears to resist extraction, occasionally grasping it with the T-handle inserter and rotating the nail will loosen it sufficiently to facilitate the procedure.

5 Suggested reading

Bar-On E, Sagiv S, Porat S (1997)
External fixation or flexible intramedullary nailing for femoral shaft fractures in children.
J Bone Joint Surg. [Br]; 79-B: 975–978.

Carey TP, Galpin RD (1996)
Flexible intramedullary nail fixation of pediatric femoral fractures.
Clin Orthop; 332:110–118.

Dietz HG, Schmittenbecher PP, Illing P (1996)
Die intramedulläre Osteosynthese im Wachstumsalter.
Urban & München-Wien-Baltimore: Schwarzenberg.

Dietz HG, Joppich I, Marzi I, et al (2001)
[Treatment of femoral fractures in childhood. Consensus Report of the 19th Meeting of the Child Traumatology Section of the DGU, Munich, 23–24 June 2000.]
Unfallchirurg; 104(8):788–790.

Hedin H (2004)
Surgical treatment of femoral fractures in children. Comparison between external fixation and elastic intramedullary nails: a review.
Acta Orthop Scand; 75(3):231–240.

Heyworth BE, Galano GJ, Vitale MA, et al (2004)
Management of closed femoral shaft fractures in children, ages 6 to 10: national practice patterns and emerging trends.
J Pediatr Orthop; 24(5):455–459.

Houshian S, Gothgen CB, Pedersen NW, et al (2004)
Femoral shaft fractures in children: elastic stable intramedullary nailing in 31 cases.
Acta Orthop Scand; 75(3):249–251.

Jubel A, Andermahr J, Prokop A, et al (2004)
[Pitfalls and complications of elastic stable intramedullary nailing (ESIN) of femoral fractures in infancy.]
Unfallchirurg; 107(9):744–749.

Ligier JN, Metaizeau JP, Prevot J, et al (1988)
Elastic stable intramedullary nailing of femoral shaft fractures in children. *J Bone Joint Surg Br;* 70(1):74–77.

Maurer G, Parsch K (2000)
Surgical Treatment of Pediatric Femoral Shaft Fractures.
Techniques in Orthopaedics; 15(1):67–78.

Metaizeau JP (2004)
Stable elastic intramedullary nailing for fractures of the femur in children.
J Bone Joint Surg Br; 86(7):954–957.

Narayanan UG, Hyman JE, Wainwright AM, et al (2004)
Complications of elastic stable intramedullary nail fixation of pediatric femoral fractures, and how to avoid them.
J Pediatr Orthop; 24(4):363–369.

Parsch KD (1997)
Modern trends in internal fixation of femoral shaft fractures in children. A critical review.
J Pediatr Orthop B; 6(2):117–125.

Schmittenbecher PP, Dietz HG (1996)
Elastic stable intramedullary nailing of femoral shaft fractures in children ("Nancy-Nailing").
Orthopaedics and Traumatology; 4201–4210.

Schmittenbecher PP, Dietz HG, Linhart WE, et al (2000)
Complications and problems in intramedullary nailing of children's fractures.
Eur J Trauma; 26(6):287–293.

Till H, Huttl B, Knorr P, et al (2000)
Elastic stable intramedullary nailing (ESIN) provides good long-term results in pediatric long-bone fractures.
Eur J Pediatr Surg; 10(5):319–322.

5.2 Proximal femoral fracture, subtrochanteric (32-D/5.1)

1 Case description

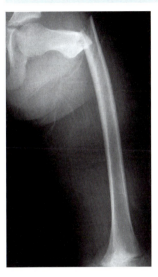

An 8-year-old boy sustained an injury to his left lower extremity while snowboarding. He presented with a markedly swollen left thigh. Clinically, this appeared to be his only injury. Distal neurovascular function was intact. X-rays taken in the emergency room revealed a displaced subtrochanteric fracture of the left femur (Fig 5.2-1). It was felt that this fracture could easily be managed by the ESIN technique and the patient was prepared for surgery.

Fig 5.2-1 The preoperative x-ray shows a high subtrochanteric fracture. A second x-ray is not needed in this case. Additional pain for the child can be avoided.

2 Surgical approach

After the left extremity has been surgically prepped and draped, bilateral symmetrical skin incisions are made (Fig 5.2-2). The distal skin landmark is the upper pole of the patella. The skin and the fascia are incised together. Blunt dissection is then continued through the muscle to the bone. Important: ensure that the entrance points are outside the joint capsule and away from the edge of the physis.

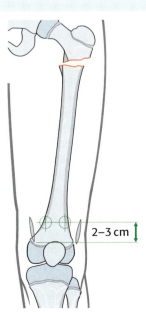

Fig 5.2-2 Skin incisions.
Symmetrical medial and lateral skin incisions start at the superior pole of the patella and progress 2–3 cm proximally.

2 Surgical approach (cont)

Entrance sites
The entry sites are first perforated by an awl in the most proximal end of the incision (2–3 cm in progress of the upper pole of the patella). The awl is initially placed 90° to the cortex to keep it from slipping off. Once the awl is firmly seated on the surface of the cortex, it is reduced to an angle of 45° to the shaft axis and the perforation of the bone is continued at an upward angle (Fig 5.2-3). If the cortex is very hard, a drill may be necessary to carefully penetrate it.

Nail selection
Determine the correct diameter of the nail by measuring the isthmus of the medullary cavity on the x-ray image. The diameter of the nail should be 1/3 of the medullary cavity at its narrowest point. Select identical nails. Using nails of different diameters can produce varus or valgus malalignment.

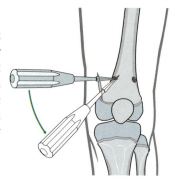

Fig 5.2-3 Awl placement. The awl is first placed perpendicular to the cortex and rotated until it is well seated in the bone. At this point it is angulated 45° to the shaft axis and advanced in order to produce a channel in the cortex.

Nail insertion
Carefully insert the nail into the medullary canal by hand or using the T-handle inserter (Fig 5.2-4). Following its insertion, the position of the nail is confirmed with the image intensifier. Note that the curve of the tip is accentuated to facilitate its bouncing off the opposite cortex. Carefully advance the first nail up to the fracture zone.

Following this, the second nail is inserted into its entrance site and advanced to the fracture zone (Fig 5.2-5).

3 Reduction and fixation

Fracture reduction
At the fracture site, one of the nails is usually manipulated in such a manner that its tip reduces the fragments (Fig 5.2-6). Once the reduction has been accomplished, both nails are advanced into the proximal fragment. In this case, the medial nail should be directed to the femoral neck and the lateral nail toward the greater trochanter. Just prior to advancing to their final position, the nails are cut leaving enough length to manipulate and advance them to their final position (Fig 5.2-7). Once both nails have entered the proximal fragment they are then tapped toward their final position (Fig 5.2-8).

Final positioning
Once the nail tips are in their final position, the end of each nail is cut, leaving 1–2 cm protruding from the cortex (Fig 5.2-9b). The amount left protruding is dependent upon the amount of soft-tissue coverage around the tips. After cutting to the final length, caps can be placed over the protruding ends of the nails to protect the soft tissues (Fig 5.2-9a).

Very proximal position
In the final reduction, the tips should be aligned so that the lateral nail tip is directed toward the greater trochanter and the medial nail tip is placed in the femoral neck almost up to the physeal plate. It needs to be emphasized here that nails stabilizing subtrochanteric fractures are passed as proximal as possible into the intertrochanteric region to provide enhanced stability. Passing the nails proximally to this degree is not necessary to stabilize midshaft fractures.

5.2 Proximal femoral fracture, subtrochanteric (32-D/5.1)

3 Reduction and fixation (cont)

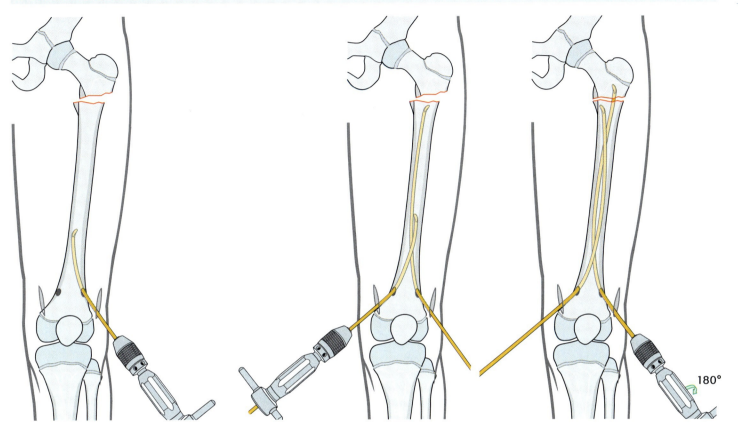

Fig 5.2-4 Insertion of first nail.
The first nail is inserted into the medullary cavity and advanced proximally. The bend in the tip may need to be increased slightly to facilitate its advancing past the opposite cortex.

Fig 5.2-5 Insertion of second nail.
Once the first nail has been advanced to the fracture site, the second nail is inserted and also advanced proximally.

Fig 5.2-6 Fracture reduction.
The tip of one of the nails is manipulated to enter the medullary canal of the proximal fragment. It is rotated (circular arrow) so as to improve the reduction.

5 Femur

3 Reduction and fixation (cont)

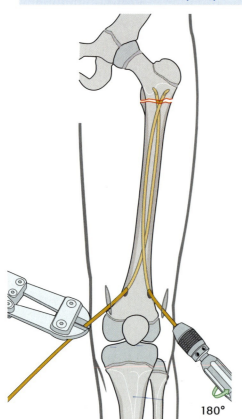

Fig 5.2-7   Proximal advancement.
Both nails are advanced into the proximal fragment with one directed into the femoral neck and the other toward the greater trochanter. A preliminary cut is made, leaving enough length for the final advancement.

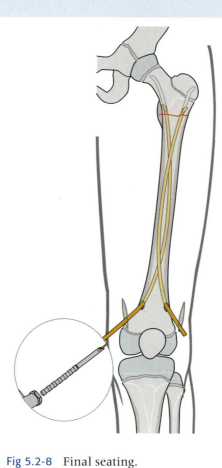

Fig 5.2-8   Final seating.
Once the correct direction and position have been established, the nails are tapped into their final position (dotted lines). One tip lies within the greater trochanter, while the other lies just distal to the capital physis.

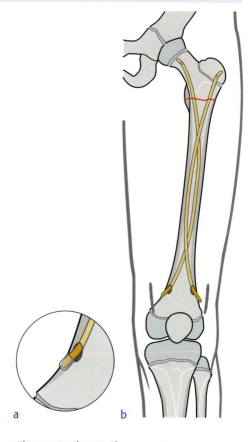

Fig 5.2-9a–b   Nail protection.
Plastic caps or end caps are placed over the cut end. The wound is closed.

5.2 Proximal femoral fracture, subtrochanteric (32-D/5.1)

4 Postoperative care and rehabilitation

Postoperatively, the child is allowed as much motion of the extremity as tolerated. They are usually mobilized without crutches. The first x-rays are taken in the outpatient clinic at 4 weeks (Fig 5.2-10). If there is sufficient callus, full weight bearing can begin. Usually there is sufficient healing by 8 months to consider removal of the nails (Fig 5.2-11).

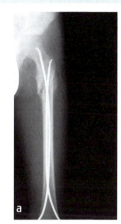 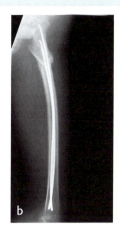 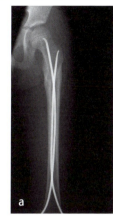 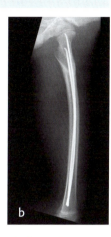

Fig 5.2-10a–b AP and lateral x-rays taken 4 weeks after ESIN demonstrate sufficient healing to allow full weight bearing.

Fig 5.2-11a–b AP and lateral x-rays taken 8 months after ESIN demonstrate sufficient consolidation to permit nail removal.

5 Pitfalls –

Approach
Making the incision too proximal.

The physis is injured by too distal insertion of the nail.

The entrance points are not on the same level.

6 Pearls +

Approach
The entrance sites need to be at a sufficient distance from the fracture site, to ensure that the fracture site is not entered or violated and remains closed.

5 Pitfalls – (cont)

Reduction and fixation
Perforation of the proximal cortex during insertion.

Corkscrew phenomenon with more than two nail junctions.

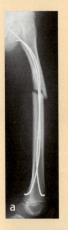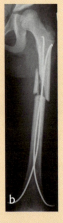

Fig 5.2-12a–b   Crossing the nails at the fracture site instead of having the maximum separation in this area.

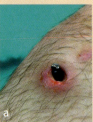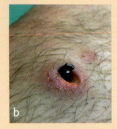

Fig 5.2-13a–b   Leaving the nails too long causes the ends to irritate the skin enough to predispose it to perforation and a subsequent infection.

6 Pearls + (cont)

Reduction and fixation—special case
A 14-year-old male was struck by a car, sustaining a subtrochanteric fracture of his right femur. 3 months earlier, he had undergone bilateral in situ screw fixation as treatment for a slipped capital femoral epiphysis. The fracture occurred at the level of the screw head (Fig 5.2-14).

Prior to the development of the ESIN technique, treatment of such a fracture would have most likely required an open procedure and the use of a large plate and/or hip screw. This fracture was easily stabilized by passing the flexible nails retrograde around the screw (Fig 5.2-14).

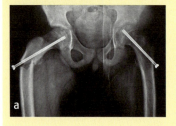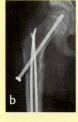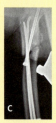

Fig 5.2-14a–c
a   The fracture appears to originate in the subtrochanteric area where the screw entered the lateral cortex.
b–c   AP and lateral x-rays show the nails passing around the screw to be secured in the proximal femur. There is early callus formation.

Rehabilitation

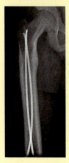

Immediate mobilization was initiated on crutches. The patient progressed to full weight bearing at 4 weeks by which time x-rays revealed good callus formation.

Fig 5.2-15   The screw was removed 1 year after the accident. X-rays 6 months after removal of the screw demonstrate that there is sufficient healing of the fracture to consider nail removal.

5.3 Femoral shaft fracture, transverse (32-D/4.1)

1 Case description

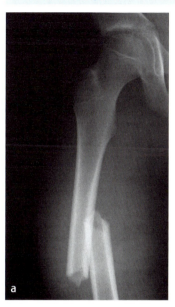
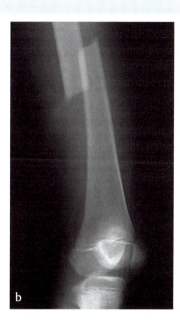

General consideration
The management of oblique and transverse fracture patterns of the femoral shaft using the ESIN technique is essentially the same. The following case describes the management of a transverse femoral midshaft fracture. An alternative case with a spiral femoral shaft fracture is presented later on in this chapter.

Case 32-D/4.1
A 10-year-old boy fell off his bicycle and presented with a markedly swollen and painful right thigh. X-rays taken in the emergency room revealed a transverse midshaft fracture of the right femur (Fig 5.3-1). The fracture was closed and presented as an isolated injury. There were no neurovascular complications.

Fig 5.3-1a–b AP and lateral x-rays showing transverse midshaft fracture of the right femur. There was significant shortening but minimal angulation.

2 Surgical approach

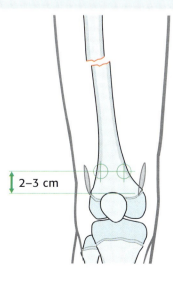

Skin incisions
After the extremity has been surgically prepped and draped, bilateral symmetrical skin incisions are made (Fig 5.3-2). The distal skin landmark is the upper pole of the patella. The skin and the fascia are incised together. Blunt dissection is then continued through the muscle to the bone. Important: ensure that the entrance points are outside the joint capsule and away from the edge of the physis.

Fig 5.3-2 Skin incisions.
Symmetrical medial and lateral skin incisions start at the superior pole of the patella and progress proximally 2–3 cm.

2 Surgical approach (cont)

Entrance site
The cortex is first perforated by an awl. It is initially placed 90° to the cortex to keep it from slipping off. Once the awl is firmly seated on the surface of the cortex, it is angled so that the entrance channel is 45° to the cortex (Fig 5.3-3). If the cortex is very hard, a drill may be necessary to carefully penetrate the cortex.

Nail selection
Determine the correct diameter of the nail by measuring the isthmus of the medullary canal on the x-ray image. The diameter of the nail should be 1/3 of the medullary canal at its narrowest point. Select identical nails. Using nails of different diameters can produce varus or valgus malalignment. A small extra bend is made at the tip to facilitate its bouncing off the opposite cortex.

Nail insertion
Carefully insert the nail into the medullary canal by hand or using the T-handle inserter(Fig 5.3-4). Initially, it is often easiest to insert the nail tip by hand. After its insertion, the position of the nail is confirmed with the image intensifier.

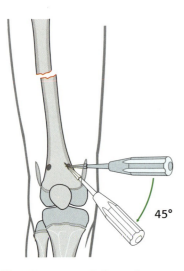

Fig 5.3-3 Placement of the awl.
The awl is first placed perpendicular to the cortex and rotated until it is well seated in the bone. At this point it is then angulated 45° to the shaft axis to produce an oblique channel in the cortex.

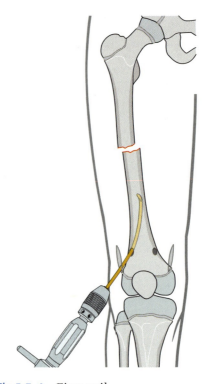

Fig 5.3-4 First nail.
The tip of the precontoured nail is inserted first into the medullary canal and advanced proximally. To facilitate its making the first turn against the opposite inner cortex, a slight curve is initially placed in the nail just proximal to the tip.

5.3 Femoral shaft fracture, transverse (32-D/4.1)

2 Surgical approach (cont)

Carefully advance the first nail toward the fracture zone. Following this, the second nail is inserted and advanced to the fracture zone (Fig 5.3-5). The order in which the nail is passed depends upon which one passes more easily.

3 Reduction and fixation

Fracture reduction

At the fracture site, one of the nails is usually manipulated in such a manner that its tip reduces the fragments. Once the reduction has been accomplished, both nails are advanced into the proximal fragment (Fig 5.3-6). In this case, the medial nail should be advanced into the femoral neck and the lateral nail toward the greater trochanter. This is not as far as for subtrochanteric fractures (see Fig 5.2-9). Just prior to advancing the nails to their final position, they are cut leaving enough length to manipulate and advance them further (see Fig 5.3-7).

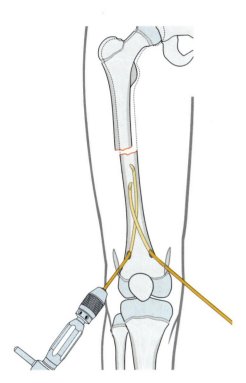

Fig 5.3-5 Second nail.
The first nail is advanced proximal to the fracture zone. Likewise, the second precontoured nail is inserted into the entrance site and advanced proximal to the fracture site.

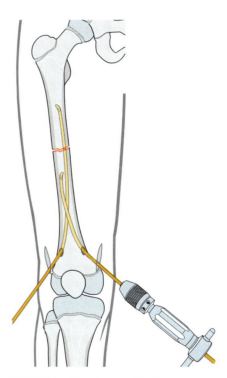

Fig 5.3-6 Fracture reduction.
Once both nails have reached the fracture site, the lateral one (the first nail inserted) is manipulated to enter the medullary canal of the proximal fragment so as to complete the reduction of the fracture. The second nail is then advanced to the proximal fragment.

3 Reduction and fixation (cont)

Final positioning

Once the nail tips are in their final position, the end of each nail is cut leaving 1–2 cm protruding from the cortex (Fig 5.3-8). The length depends on the amount of soft-tissue coverage around the tips. After cutting to the final length, caps are placed over the protruding ends of the nails to protect the soft tissues.

In the final reduction the tips should be aligned so that the lateral nail tip is directed toward the greater trochanter and the medial nail tip is directed toward the neck of the femur. Note that the final location of the nail tips for stabilizing shaft fractures is no further than the level of the most proximal portion of the lesser trochanter.

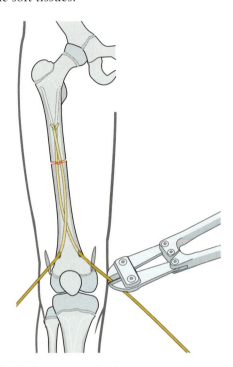

Fig 5.3-7 Proximal advancement.
The ends of the nails are first cut leaving sufficient length to continue their easy passage proximally. Enough length is left so that the tips can be advanced to just above the level of the lesser trochanter (dotted nail tips). For most shaft fractures advancement of the tips to the level of the lesser trochanter is usually sufficient.

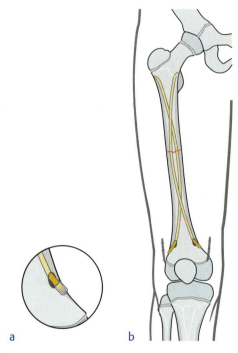

Fig 5.3-8a–b Nail protection.
Once the nails are in their final position they are cut again leaving only 1–2 cm protruding outside the cortex. Plastic caps or end caps are placed over the cut end. The wound is closed.

5.3 Femoral shaft fracture, transverse (32-D/4.1)

4 Postoperative care and rehabilitation

Postoperative x-rays (Fig 5.3-9) demonstrate satisfactory positioning of the nails with the tips just proximal to the lesser trochanter. There is good separation of the nails in the fracture zone. Protected weight bearing can be allowed.

By 3 months postoperatively a proliferative callus has developed around the fracture site (Fig 5.3-10). X-rays taken at 8 months postoperatively following nail removal demonstrate complete remodeling of the initial callus (Fig 5.3-11).

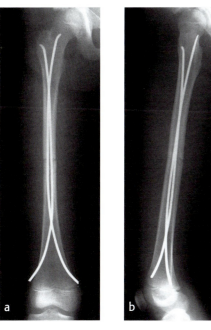

Fig 5.3-9a–b AP and lateral x-rays postoperatively demonstrate optimal positioning of the nails. The tips are just proximal to the lesser trochanter. There is good separation in the fracture zone.

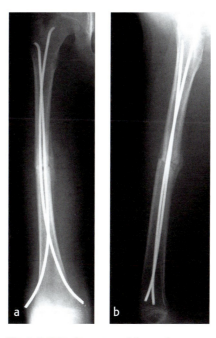

Fig 5.3-10a–b AP and lateral x-rays taken at 3 months demonstrate good callus surrounding the fracture site.

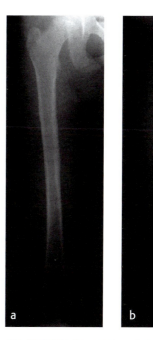

Fig 5.3-11a–b AP and lateral x-rays taken 8 months after nail removal with complete remodeling of the callus.

5 Alternative case—unstable oblique/spiral femoral shaft fracture (32-D/5.1)

Even in long, unstable spiral fractures, ESIN can be used. To prevent the danger of shortening correct application of the proper technique is mandatory.

Especially:
- respect of biomechanics
- entry points
- nail positioning and placing
- prebending of nails

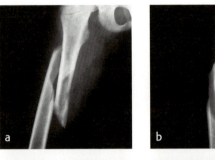

A 10-year-old boy fell while skating and presented to the emergency room with a swollen right thigh as his only injury. X-rays revealed a spiral fracture of the midshaft of his right femur.

Fig 5.3-12a–b   AP and lateral injury x-rays demonstrating a long spiral midshaft fracture of his right femur with only moderate shortening.

The patient was taken to surgery and the femur was stabilized using the ESIN technique in exactly the same manner as described in the previous case (see Figs 5.3-1 to 5.3-9). Postoperative x-rays demonstrate a good anatomical reduction and fixation.

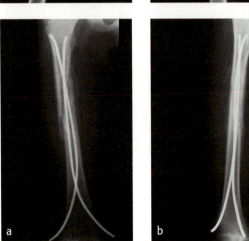

Fig 5.3-13a–b   AP and lateral x-rays at 2 weeks postoperatively showing the fracture reduced and excellent separation of the tension bends of the nails at the fracture site.

The boy was permitted full postoperative mobilization. In this case mobilization was facilitated by the use of a continuous passive motion machine (CPM) immediately after surgery. CPM is not used routinely. It is useful in those patients who are slow in initiating their postoperative motion.

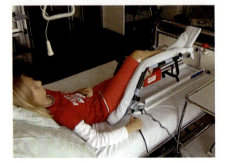

Fig 5.3-14   Reestablishment of motion can be facilitated with the use of CPM.

5.3 Femoral shaft fracture, transverse (32-D/4.1)

5 Alternative case—unstable oblique/spiral femoral shaft fracture (32-D/5.1) (cont)

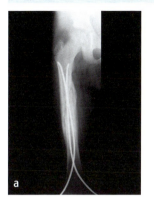
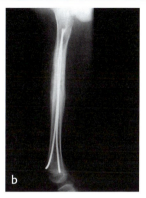

Fig 5.3-15a–b   Proliferative callus. The x-rays at 3 months show a stabilized fracture with abundant callus. There is also early remodeling.

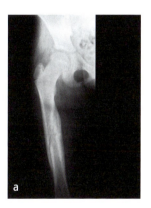
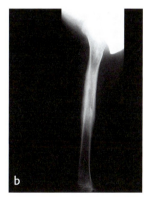

Fig 5.3-16a–b   Complete recovery. 8 months after nail removal, the patient is fully active with no leg length discrepancy. X-rays demonstrate complete remodeling of the fracture.

6 Pitfalls –

Approach

Fig 5.3-17   The incision is too proximal and too small. If the incision is placed too proximal, the oblique angle of insertion may cause the awl to injure the distal end of the incision. This could result in local necrosis with a subsequent infection.

7 Pearls +

Approach

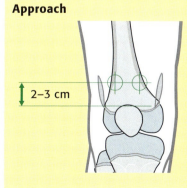

Fig 5.3-18   Proper location of the incision. Symmetrical medial and lateral skin incisions start at the superior poles of the patella and progress proximally 2–3 cm.

6 Pitfalls − (cont)

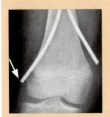

Fig 5.3-19 The entrance point is directly adjacent to the physis. If this is the case, the periphery of the physis can be injured during drilling in an oblique direction. Hence, the distal entrance sites should be 1–2 cm proximal to the edge of the physis.

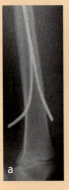 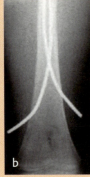

Fig 5.3-20a–b The entrance points are not on the same level.
If the entrance points are at different levels, the nails may have unequal tension forces. This can result in the development of angular deformities.

Reduction and fixation
Perforation of the opposite cortex.
If the nail is not advanced in an oblique direction during insertion, it can easily penetrate the thin cortex of the opposing side of the metaphysis.

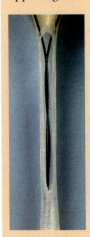

Fig 5.3-21 Corkscrew phenomenon. Never turn the nail on its own axis by more than 180°, as this produces more than two nail junctions or the "corkscrew phenomenon". This configuration effectively eliminates the stabilizing effects of the nails.

7 Pearls + (cont)

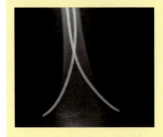

Fig 5.3-22 The entrance points are on the same level.

Reduction and fixation

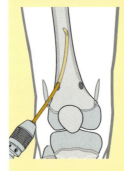

Fig 5.3-23 Oblique entrance canals. The entrance canal needs to be directed obliquely. The tip can be made to bounce off the opposite metaphyseal cortex by effecting a second curve just proximal to the one at the tip.

It is important to always follow the path of the nail tip. If there is difficulty in advancing the nail, rotate one nail under image intensifier control. Do not force the nail with the hammer if advancing it proximally is difficult. It is always best to locate the position of the tip to see if it is wedged against some obstruction.

5.3 Femoral shaft fracture, transverse (32-D/4.1)

6 Pitfalls – (cont)

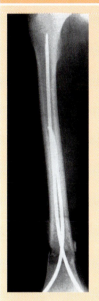

Fig 5.3-24 Crossing the nails at the fracture site.
If the nails are not spread at the fracture site, they do not exert tension forces on the fracture fragments and, thus, much of the internal stability is lost.

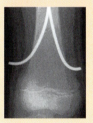

Fig 5.3-25 Leaving the ends of the nails too long can irritate the skin and block the movement of the knee.

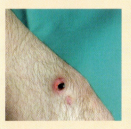

Fig 5.3-26 This skin irritation can progress to full perforation and wound infection.

7 Pearls + (cont)

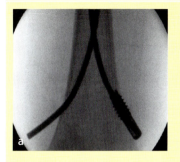 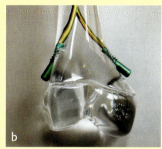

Fig 5.3-27a–b Soft tissues are best protected by using end caps.

If the end is too prominent, pull the nail back and recut it, reimplant it, or replace it.

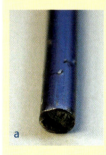 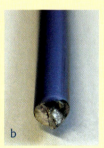

Fig 5.3-28a–b Shape of different cutted nails.
a Nail ends are cutted with the special nail cutter.
b Sharpe nail ends are cutted with a normal nail cutter.

5 Femur

5.4 Femoral shaft refracture, oblique (32-D/5.1)

1 Case description

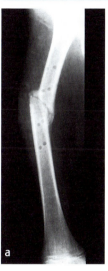
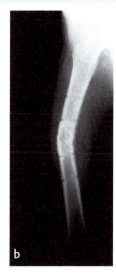

A 7-year-old boy was involved in a motor vehicle accident in which he sustained an oblique fracture of the midshaft of his right femur. He was treated immediately following that primary injury with an external fixator. This initial fracture healed uneventfully, and the fixator was removed at 10 weeks postfracture. He appeared to be progressing as expected when at 4 weeks following the removal of the fixator he jumped from a chair and fell, sustaining a new injury to his right lower extremity. X-rays taken in the emergency room demonstrated a refracture through the old fracture site (Fig 5.4-1). Commonly, femoral fractures treated with an external fixator show poor callus at the old fracture site. This is felt to be due to the stress shielding from the fixator.

Fig 5.4-1a–b Injury x-rays, taken immediately post-refracture. In addition to varus angulation, the distal fragment is also internally rotated and there is poor callus.

2 Surgical approach

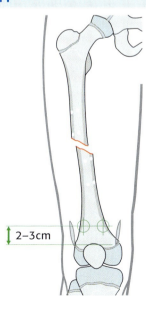

The surgical approach is very similar to the one used for the primary fractures of the femoral shaft following the standard ESIN technique for femoral shaft fractures.

After the extremity has been surgically prepped and draped, bilateral symmetrical incisions are made (Fig 5.4-2). The distal skin landmark is the upper pole of the patella. The skin and the fascia are incised together. Blunt dissection is then continued through the muscle to the bone. Important: ensure that the entrance points are outside the joint capsule and away from the edge of the physis.

Fig 5.4-2 Skin incisions.
Symmetrical medial and lateral skin incisions start at the superior pole of the patella and progress 2–3 cm proximally.

2 Surgical approach (cont)

Cortical penetration
The cortex is first perforated by an awl. It is initially placed 90° to the cortex to keep it from slipping off. Once the awl is firmly seated on the surface of the cortex, it is angled so that the entrance channel is 45° to the cortex (Fig 5.4-3). If the cortex is very hard, a drill may be necessary to carefully penetrate the cortex.

Nail selection
Determine the correct diameter of the nail by measuring the isthmus of the medullary canal on the x-ray image. The diameter of the nail should be 1/3 of the medullary canal at its narrowest point. It is important to select identical nails. Using nails of different diameters creates unequal tension leading to varus or valgus malalignment. A small extra bend is made at the tip to facilitate its bouncing off the opposite cortex.

Nail insertion
Carefully insert the first nail into the medullary canal by hand or by using the inserter (Fig 5.4-4). Initially, it is often easiest to insert the nail tip by hand. After its insertion, the position of the nail is confirmed with the image intensifier.

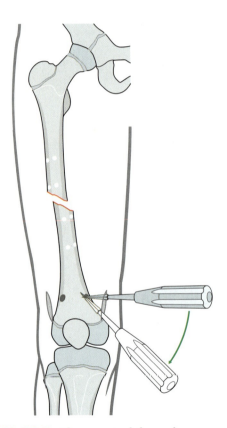

Fig 5.4-3 Placement of the awl.
The awl is first placed perpendicular to the cortex and rotated until it is well seated in the bone. At this point, it is then angulated 45° to the shaft axis to produce an oblique channel in the cortex.

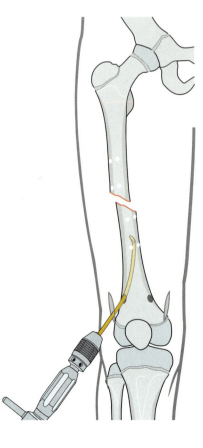

Fig 5.4-4 First nail.
The tip of the precontoured nail is inserted first into the medullary canal and advanced proximally. To facilitate its making the first turn against the opposite inner cortex, a slight curve is initially made in the nail just proximal to the tip.

5.4 Femoral shaft refracture, oblique (32-D/5.1)

2 Surgical approach (cont)

Carefully advance the first nail toward the fracture zone. Following this, the second nail is inserted into its entrance site and advanced to the fracture zone (Fig 5.4-5). The order in which the nails are passed depends upon which one passes more easily.

3 Reduction and fixation

Fracture reduction
At the fracture site, one of the nails is usually manipulated in such a manner that its tip reduces the fragments. Once the reduction has been accomplished, both nails are advanced into the proximal fragment (Fig 5.4-6). In this case, the medial nail should be advanced into the femoral neck and the lateral nail toward the greater trochanter. This is not as far as with subtrochanteric fractures (see Fig 5.2-7). Just prior to advancing the nails to their final position, they are cut (Fig 5.4-7), leaving enough length to manipulate and advance them further.

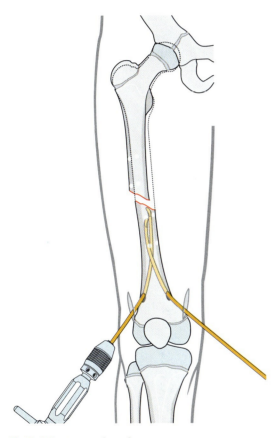

Fig 5.4-5 Second nail.
The first nail is advanced proximally to the fracture zone. Likewise, the second precontoured nail is inserted into the entrance site and advanced proximally to the fracture site.

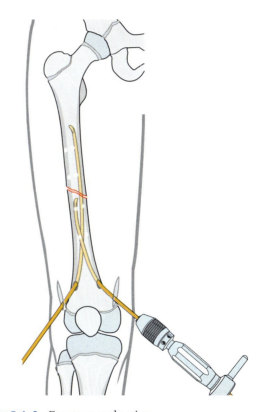

Fig 5.4-6 Fracture reduction.
Once both nails have reached the fracture site, one of them is manipulated to enter the medullary canal of the proximal fragment and to complete the reduction of the fracture. Both nails are then advanced proximally into the proximal fragment.

5 Femur

3 Reduction and fixation (cont)

Final positioning
Once the nail tips are in their final position, the end of each nail is cut leaving 1–2 cm protruding from the cortex (Fig 5.4-8). The amount left protruding is dependent upon the amount of soft-tissue coverage around the tips. After cutting to the final length, caps are placed over the protruding ends of the nails to protect the soft tissues.

Tips diverge
In the final reduction the tips should be aligned so that the lateral nail tip is directed toward the greater trochanter and the medial nail tip is directed toward the neck of the femur (Fig 5.4-8). Note that the final location of the tips of the nails for stabilizing shaft fractures is advanced only up to the level of the most proximal portion of the lesser trochanter.

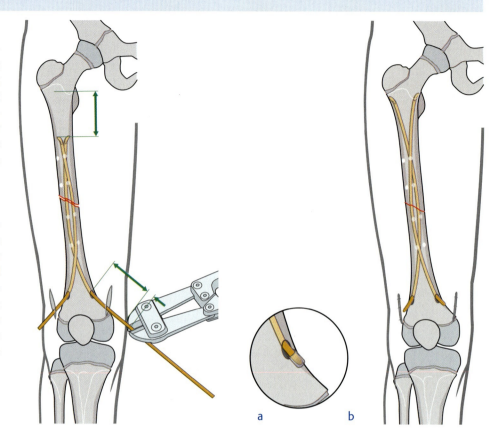

Fig 5.4-7 Primary nail cutting.
The ends of the nails are first cut, leaving sufficient length to continue their easy passage proximally. Enough length is left so that the tips can be advanced to just above the level of the lesser trochanter. For most shaft fractures advancement of the tips to this level is usually sufficient.

Fig 5.4-8a–b Nail protection.
Once the nails have been advanced to their final position, they are cut again leaving only 1–2 cm protruding outside the cortex. Plastic caps or end caps are placed over the cut end. The wound is closed.

5.4 Femoral shaft refracture, oblique (32-D/5.1)

4 Postoperative care and rehabilitation

Because of the stability of the fracture following ESIN, the patient can begin immediate mobilization progressing rapidly to weight bearing as tolerated using crutches.

The first follow-up x-rays are usually taken at about 2–4 weeks postoperatively.

The position of the fractures and nails should be unchanged. Depending upon the original severity of the fracture and rate of return of motion and muscle strength, the child is seen at the appropriate intervals. Once the fracture has healed and the callus has remodeled (Fig 5.4-9), the child is scheduled for nail removal.

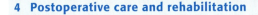

Fig 5.4-9a–b AP and lateral x-rays taken at 8 months postoperatively demonstrate obliteration of the fracture line and the defects from the fixator pins.

5 Femur

5.5 Segmental femoral shaft fracture (32-D/5.2) and ipsilateral tibial shaft fracture (42-D/5.1)

1 Case description

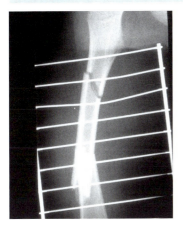

Fig 5.5-1 Femoral fracture. The fractures are oblique and transverse and are located at the junctions of the proximal-middle and middle-distal segments of the shaft.

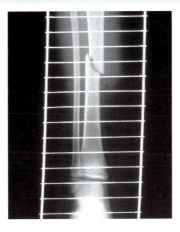

Fig 5.5-2 Tibial fracture. The ipsilateral facture of the tibia is an isolated oblique fracture pattern located in the mid-shaft.

A 7-year-old boy injured in a car-pedestrian accident presented with multiple system injuries. His life-threatening conditions included a closed head injury and blunt trauma to the chest.

The patient's major orthopedic concerns included a segmental fracture of the right femoral shaft with shortening (Fig 5.5-1). Additionally, he suffered from an oblique fracture of the midshaft of the ipsilateral tibia which was only minimally displaced and shortened (Fig 5.5-2).

In this case of polytrauma and under the aspect of primary care and rehabilitation the isolated tibial shaft fracture has to be operated too.

Initial stabilization
The patient's potentially life-threatening conditions were evaluated with CT scans of the head and thorax. In addition, a tube was inserted into one of the ventricles to monitor for increases in the intraventricular pressure. Fortunately, these initial evaluations demonstrated that he had no life-threatening conditions and was neurologically and hemodynamically stable.

Femur stabilized initially
Once it was determined that the boy was stable enough to be anesthetized, he was transferred to the operating room and was positioned supine on a radiolucent operating table. It was elected to stabilize the femur first.

Convert to two segments
The basic principle in treating a segmental fracture is to first convert it to two workable segments. An evaluation of the pattern and location of the fractures will determine which segments should be connected first. This same evaluation will also determine whether the nailing procedure should be performed ante- or retrograde.

Retrograde nailing
In this patient, because there was only a relatively short amount of cortex proximally, it was felt that the stabilization could be best performed in retrograde technique.

2 Surgical approach

Skin incisions

After the extremity has been surgically prepped and draped, bilateral symmetrical incisions are made (Fig 5.5-3). The distal skin landmark is the upper pole of the patella. The skin and the fascia are incised together. Blunt dissection is then continued through the muscle to the bone. Important: Ensure that the entrance points are outside the joint capsule and away from the edge of the physis.

Cortical penetration

The cortex is first perforated by an awl. It is initially placed 90° to the cortex to keep it from slipping off. Once the awl is firmly seated on the surface of the cortex, it is angled so that the entrance channel is 45° to the cortex (Fig 5.5-4). If the cortex is very hard, a drill may be necessary to carefully penetrate the cortex.

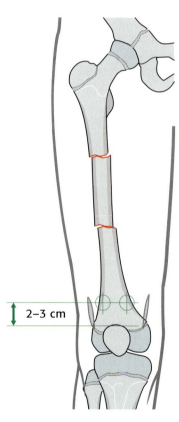

Fig 5.5-3 Skin incisions.
Symmetrical medial and lateral skin incisions start at the superior pole of the patella and progress 2–3 cm proximally.

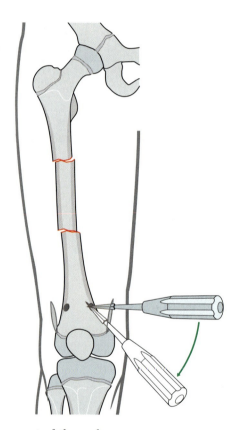

Fig 5.5-4 Placement of the awl.
The awl is first placed perpendicular to the cortex and rotated until it is well seated in the bone. At this point, it is then angulated 45° to the shaft axis to produce an oblique channel in the cortex.

5.5 Segmental femoral shaft fracture (32-D/5.2) and ipsilateral tibial shaft fracture (42-D/5.1)

2 Surgical approach (cont)

Nail selection

Determine the correct diameter of the nail by measuring the isthmus of the medullary canal on the x-ray image. The diameter of the nail should be 1/3 of the medullary canal at its narrowest point. It is important to select identical nails. Using nails of different diameters creates unequal tensions leading to varus or valgus malalignment. A small extra bend is made at the tip to facilitate its bouncing off the opposite cortex.

Nail insertion

Carefully insert the nail into the medullary canal by hand or by using the T-handle inserter (Fig 5.5-5). Initially it is often easiest to insert the nail tip by hand. After its insertion, the position of the nail is confirmed with the image intensifier.

Carefully advance the first nail toward the distal fracture zone. Following this, the second nail is inserted into its entrance site and advanced to the same fracture zone. The order in which the nails are passed depends upon which one passes more easily.

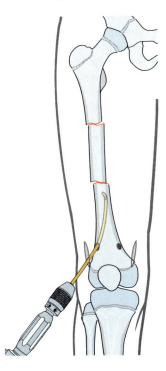

Fig 5.5-5 First nail insertion. The tip of the precontoured nail is inserted first into the medullary canal and advanced proximally. To facilitate its making the first turn against the opposite inner cortex, a slight curve is placed in the nail just proximal to the tip.

3 Reduction and fixation

Distal fracture reduction

At the fracture site, one of the nails is manipulated in such a manner that its tip reduces the distal fragment to the middle fragment. Once both nails have reached the distal fracture site, the first nail is then advanced up to the proximal fracture site (Fig 5.5-6).

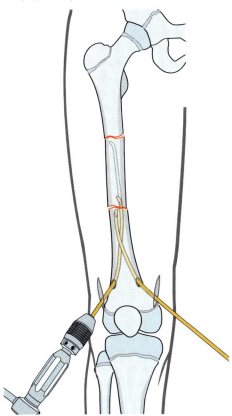

Fig 5.5-6 Distal fracture reduction. This first nail is advanced proximally to the distal fracture zone. Likewise, the second precontoured nail is inserted into its entrance site and advanced proximally to the same fracture zone. Next, the first nail is advanced to the proximal fracture zone. Once both nails have reached the fracture site, one of them is manipulated to enter the medullary canal of the proximal fragment and manipulated so as to complete the reduction of the fracture.

5 Femur

3 Reduction and fixation   (cont)

Once this first reduction has been achieved, the second nail is advanced fully into the middle fragment (Fig 5.5-7).

Proximal fracture reduction
The three-segment fracture has now been converted to two segments. A second indirect fracture reduction is again accomplished by manipulation of one of the nail tips and by advancing it into the most proximal fragment (Fig 5.5-8).

First nail cuts
Once this secondary reduction has been achieved, the second nail is then advanced into the proximal fragment. The excess part of the nail is first trimmed leaving only an amount protruding equal to the distance needed to advance to the final position plus the 1–1.5 cm that will be left protruding from the cortex (Fig 5.5-9).

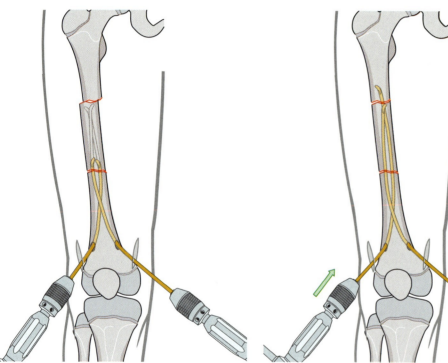
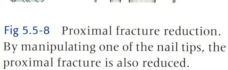
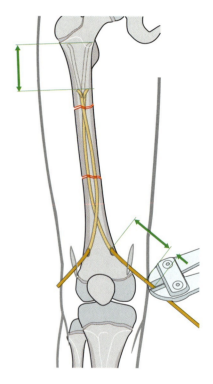

Fig 5.5-7 Middle segment stabilization.
The middle segment is stabilized to the distal segment as both nails are then advanced proximally into the central fragment to the proximal fracture zone.

Fig 5.5-8 Proximal fracture reduction. By manipulating one of the nail tips, the proximal fracture is also reduced.

Fig 5.5-9 Nail cutting.
The ends of the nails are first cut, leaving sufficient length to continue their easy passage proximally. Enough length is left so that the tips can be advanced into the proximal fragment to just above the level of the lesser trochanter. For most shaft fractures, advancement of the tips to this level is usually sufficient.

5.5 Segmental femoral shaft fracture (32-D/5.2) and ipsilateral tibial shaft fracture (42-D/5.1)

3 Reduction and fixation (cont)

Final advancement
Both nails are now ready to be advanced into the proximal fragment. In this case, the medial nail should be advanced into the femoral neck and the lateral nail towards the greater trochanter.

Final positioning
Nail cutting.
Once the nail tips are in their final position, the end of each nail is then cut, leaving 1–2 cm. protruding from the cortex (Fig 5.5-10). The amount left protruding is dependent upon the amount of soft-tissue coverage around the tips. After cutting to the final length, caps are placed over the protruding ends of the nails to protect the soft tissues.

Tips diverge
In the final reduction the tips should be aligned so that the lateral nail tip is directed towards the greater trochanter and the medial nail tip is directed toward the femoral neck. Note that the final location of the tips of the nails for stabilizing shaft fractures is no further than the level of the most proximal portion of the lesser trochanter. This is not as far as with subtrochanteric fractures (see Fig 5.2-10).

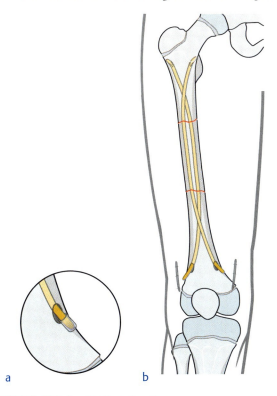

Fig 5.5-10a–b Nail protection.
Once the nails have been advanced to their final position, they are cut one last time, leaving only 1–2 cm protruding outside the cortex. Plastic caps or end caps are placed over the cut end. The wound is closed.

5 Femur

4 Stabilization of the ipsilateral tibial shaft fracture

Following the successful stabilization of the segmental femoral fracture, the tibia is stabilized using the ESIN technique described in chapter 6. The nails are inserted and advanced antegrade via separate medial and lateral entrance sites (Fig 5.5-11).

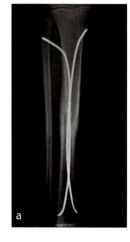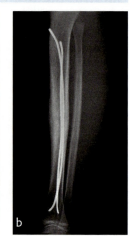

Fig 5.5-11a–b   AP and lateral follow-up x-rays of the tibia demonstrating full healing of the tibial shaft fracture following ESIN management. In this case the lateral nail has not been cut short enough.

5 Postoperative care and rehabilitation

Because of his polytrauma, this young patient remained in the ICU for a total of 3 weeks. The postoperative x-rays demonstrated that the anatomical reduction was maintained even though there was external immobilization. The patient underwent passive motion by the therapists during that time.

By week 4 there was sufficient callus visible on the x-rays of both fractures to permit full weight bearing (Fig 5.5-12).

At 8 months post-injury, the patient had regained full recovery of his muscle strength and remodeling of the fracture callus (Fig 5.5-13) to schedule nail removal.

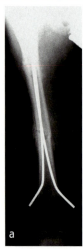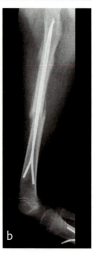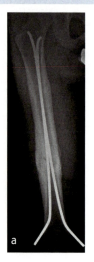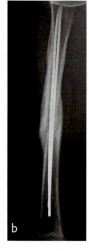

Fig 5.5-12a–b   AP and lateral x-rays 4 weeks postoperatively.

Fig 5.5-13a–b   AP and lateral x-rays at 8 months demonstrate sufficient remodeling to permit nail removal.

5.6 Distal femoral fracture (33-M/3.1)

1 Case description

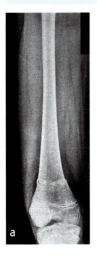
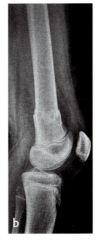
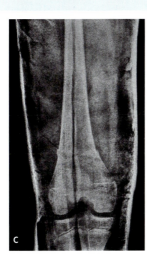
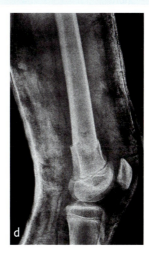

13-year-old male fell while skiing. He presented at the hospital with a temporary spica cast. X-rays taken in the emergency room showed a transverse distal femoral fracture (Fig 5.6-1).

Fig 5.6-1a–d Transverse fracture of the distal femur.

2 Surgical approach

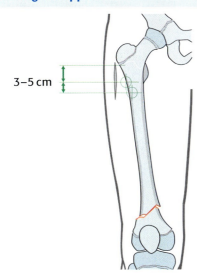

Antegrade approach
This fracture pattern is best stabilized with the ESIN technique using an antegrade approach. Thus the entrance points need to be in the proximal femur.

Skin incision
Make a 3–5 cm skin incision in the lateral aspect of the subtrochanteric region (Fig 5.6-2). The incision needs to extend proximally from the entrance sites to allow sufficient space to be able to advance the nails antegrade at an angle to the cortex. Next, spread the fascia and muscle to expose the anterolateral cortex of the femur distal to the greater trochanter.

Fig 5.6-2 Skin incision.
The proximal skin incision starts just below the greater trochanter and extends distally 3–4 cm to just below the lesser trochanter. It needs to be sufficient to allow enough exposure of the proximal shaft to accomodate the two separate entrance sites (small circles).

2 Surgical approach (cont)

Entrance sites

Two separate entrance sites 2–3 cm apart are made in the lateral cortex. Be careful, if the entrance sites are too close, the cortex may split during insertion of the nails. The entrance site is made with the awl. It is first started perpendicular to the cortex. Once it has engaged, the awl is directed at a 45° angle and drilling is continued in this direction to complete the canal in the cortex (Fig 5.6-3). These entrance canals need to be directed about 45° distally to facilitate antegrade advancement of the nails.

Nail insertion

The first nail, which has been precontoured in its distal 1/3rd, is inserted into the intramedullary canal and advanced antegrade towards the fracture site (Fig 5.6-4).

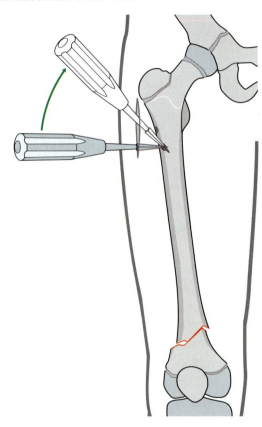

Fig 5.6-3 Entrance sites.
Once engaged, the awl is directed 45° to the shaft axis to facilitate antegrade advancement of the nails.

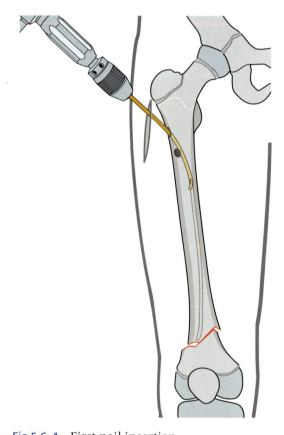

Fig 5.6-4 First nail insertion.
The first nail is inserted and advanced antegrade.

5.6 Distal femoral fracture (33-M/3.1)

3 Reduction and fixation

The second nail which is initially contoured the same as the first is then inserted into the second entrance site antegrade as well. Once it has good contact with the opposite cortex, with the tip having advanced about 2/3rds distally in the medullary canal, the contouring of the nail is ready to be changed to an S-shape (Fig 5.6-5). This is accomplished by first rotating the nail 180°. To complete the S contouring, the proximal portion of the nail still outside the entrance site is bent in a distal direction by almost 90° (Fig 5.6-6). This will convert the nail to a S-shape which will provide perfect inner contact with the lateral cortex at the fracture site and the medial cortex of the proximal femur.

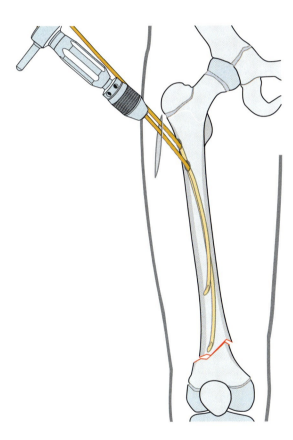

Fig 5.6-5 Second nail insertion.
The second nail is advanced until there is good contact between it and the medial cortex along the length of its curvature.

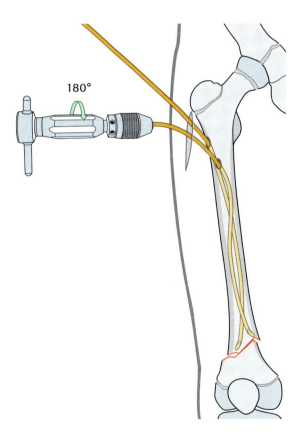

Fig 5.6-6 S-shape contouring.
The nail is first rotated 180° placing the original contour curve in contact with the lateral cortex. The portion of the nail still outside the entrance site is then bent distally by about 90°.

3 Reduction and fixation (cont)

Distal fragment advancement
If the fracture is reduced both nail tips are then advanced past the fracture site into the distal fragment (Fig 5.6-7).

Final seating
Advance the nails to the epiphyseal plate where they are impacted medially and laterally into their respective condylar regions (Fig 5.6-8a). At this time it is important to align the nail tips so that they diverge from one another. If the fracture is very distal, the physis can be perforated with the nails. It has been our experience that this does not produce any growth arrest (Fig 5.6-8b). Cut the ends and protect the soft tissue with caps (Fig 5.6-8c).

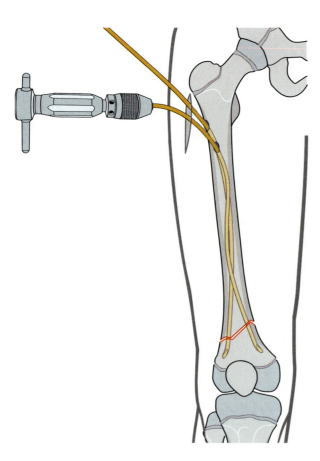

Fig 5.6-7   Distal advancement.
Once the fracture is reduced, both nails are advanced into the distal fragment.

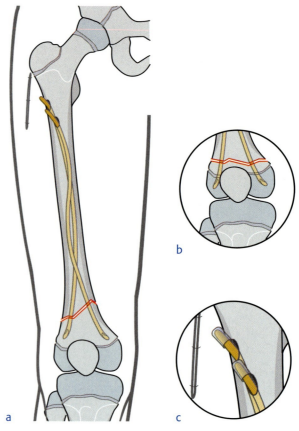

Fig 5.6-8a–c   Final seating.
After the tips have reached their final position, they are impacted into the distal fragment and cut off proximally. Plastic caps or end caps are placed over the cut end. The wound is closed.

5.6 Distal femoral fracture (33-M/3.1)

4 Postoperative care and rehabilitation

The postoperative course was uncomplicated. Because of the stability afforded by ESIN, the patient was able to initiate early motion almost immediately postoperatively.

The postoperative x-rays show anatomically reduction (Fig 5.6-9). Weight bearing with crutches was initiated as soon as the immediate postoperative pain had subsided. X-rays at 2 days and 2 weeks showed unchanged alignment (Figs 5.6-10 and 5.6-11). The ability to resume early motion enabled him to hasten his overall recovery. At 6 weeks good bone healing was visible (Fig. 5.6-12). The nails were removed at 1 year, by 2 years only 4 mm of length discrepancy and full knee motion was found.

This ability to resume early motion enabled him to hasten his overall recovery. The nails were removed at one year. By 2 years the x-rays demonstrated full remodeling with only 4 mm of length discrepancy and full knee motion (Fig 5.6-10).

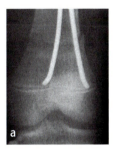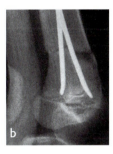

Fig 5.6-9a–b AP and lateral x-rays taken immediately after surgery. The reduction has almost obliterated the original fracture line. The nail tips lie divergently.

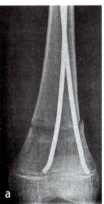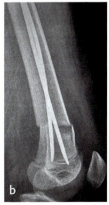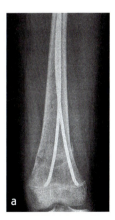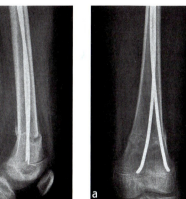

Fig 5.6-10a–b Postoperative x-rays after 2 days show correct axial alignment of the fracture.

Fig 5.6-11a–b Follow-up x-rays after 2 weeks show good remodeling of the bone.

Fig 5.6-12a–b Follow-up x-rays after 6 weeks show good bone healing.

5 Pitfalls −

Approach
Retrograde nail may produce an unstable construct.

Reduction and fixation
Because of the need for separation of the entrance sites proximally, the nail lengths are unequal. Therefore, there needs to be an anatomical reduction.

6 Pearls +

Approach
The proximal approach produces only minimal scaring.

Reduction and fixation
If the fracture is unstable due to comminution, a small external fixator can be applied to maintain length temporarily.

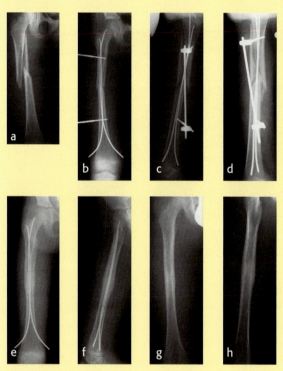

Fig 5.6-13a–h
a   Multifragmentary fracture in osteoporotic bone.
b   ESIN with additional small external fixator, AP view.
c   ESIN with additional small external fixator, lateral view.
d   The external fixator can be removed if callus is visible.
e   Healing after 3 months, AP view.
f   Healing after 3 months, lateral view.
g   Follow-up after 1 year, AP view.
h   Follow-up after 1 year, lateral view.

5.6 Distal femoral fracture (33-M/3.1)

5 Pitfalls – (cont)

Reduction and fixation (cont)

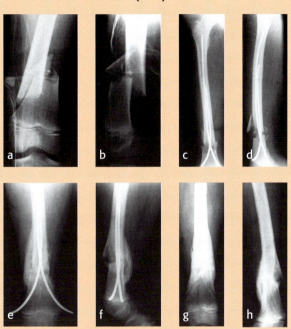

5.6-14a–h Unstable construct.
a–b A 14 year-old-male was involved in an car-pedestrian accident. On presentation to the emergency room, his only physical finding was a swollen right thigh. X-rays demonstrated a completely displaced transverse fracture through the distal femur at the diaphyseal-metaphyseal junction.
c–d He was treated with ESIN using a retrograde approach.
e–f This, however, was not a stable construct. Because the entrance sites were close to the fracture site the nails crossed at the fracture site providing very little intrinsic stability. As a result he required external immobilization which delayed the onset of early motion resulting in a prolonged postoperative rehabilitation period.
g–h Fortunately, his fracture progressed to full healing.

6 Pearls + (cont)

Reduction and fixation (cont)

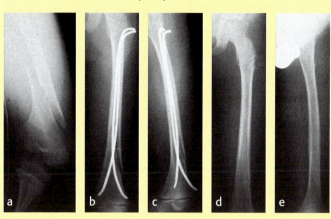

Fig 5.6-15a–e An 8-year-old boy fell while skiing and presented with a painful and swollen left thigh.
This was an isolated injury. X-rays revealed an oblique fracture of the distal left femur.
a Oblique fracture of the distal femur.
b–c AP and lateral x-rays taken immediately following the surgery. The reduction has almost obliterated the original fracture line. The nail tips lie divergently.
d–e Complete remodeling. AP and lateral x-rays taken 2 years post-fracture demonstrate complete remodeling of the fracture site.

6 Tibia

6.1 Introduction—tibial fractures 149
 1 Indications 149
 2 Patient preparation and positioning 149
 3 Surgical principle 150
 4 Implant removal 150
 5 Suggested reading 150

6.2 Tibial and fibular midshaft fracture, oblique (42-D/5.1) 151

6.3 Isolated tibial shaft fracture, oblique (42t-D/5.1) 157

6.4 Tibial midshaft fracture, wedge (42t-D/5.2) 163

6.1 Introduction—tibial fractures

1 Indications

Some fractures of the tibia have an acceptable alignment and can be immobilized simply with a plaster cast. Those fractures which may require a manipulation to achieve an acceptable alignment prior to their being immobilized can present with one of the following conditions:
- Ante- or recurvature > 10°.
- Lateral displacement exceeding 1/2 the diameter of the shaft.
- Varus or valgus angulation > 10°.
- Shortening.
- Rotational malalignment.
- Malalignment of up to 10° can be immobilized initially with a plaster cast followed by corrective wedging of the cast after 1 week.

Operative indications
While a large number of fractures of the tibia can be managed quite adequately by nonoperative methods, there are certain situations in which operative intervention must be employed to achieve an acceptable result. The indications for surgical management include:
- Unstable fractures of the distal shaft including the adjacent distal metaphysis.
- Irreducible fractures.
- Unstable fractures in which a satisfactory alignment can not be maintained by external immobilization alone.
- Gustilo type II and III open fractures.
- Fractures associated with vessel and/or nerve injuries.

The triangular shape of the tibial head, the two lateral planes tilted forwards, and the remote medullary cavity mean that nails can not be inserted laterally as in the femur. To prevent recurvation of the tibial shaft caused by the dorsal movement of the nail apexes, nails must be inserted at a specific point with the apexes rotated dorsally.
Moreover, the fact that the tibia is asymmetrical in relation to the associated musculature often leads to malunion or nonunion.

Isolated tibial shaft fractures
With some fractures of the tibial shaft, the fibula may remain intact. If this occurs, the force of the gastrocnemius-soleus complex is converted from one of simple shortening to one of rotation. This change in direction of the muscle force can result in the tibia developing varus angulation. If this varus malalignment shifts into more than 10°, it can be managed only by operative intervention. Persistence of this malalignment can prolong the healing time and present an increased risk for the development of pseudarthrosis.

2 Patient preparation and positioning

Medication
Antibiotic prophylaxis is administered according to the standard of care in the local community. Thrombosis prophylaxis is usually indicated for menstruating girls, overweight patients and patients with pelvic injuries.

Equipment
In addition to the usual surgical instruments needed for most orthopedic procedures, some special equipment is essential. This includes:
- Standard ESIN set
- Nails:
  2.0–4.0 mm stainless steel or titanium; 33% (1/3) of the medullary canal of the tibial shaft at its narrowest point.
- Image intensifier

2 Patient preparation and positioning (cont)

Patient positioning
The child is placed in the supine position with a support placed under the knee (Fig 6.1-1). It is important to ensure that leg lengths can be compared with each other at the end of the operation.

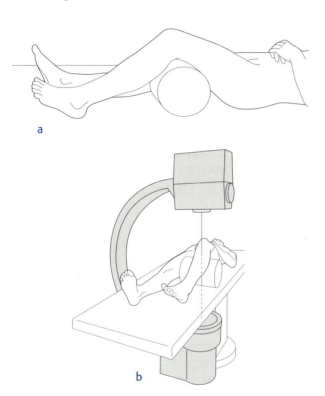

Fig 6.1-1a–b   Positioning of the limb.
a   The injured leg is supported with a holding device so that both the AP and lateral images can be easily obtained without much movement of the extremity.
b   The image intensifier is placed with enough space to allow its rotation to obtain a true AP image of the tibia.

3 Surgical principle

Direction of nailing
These fractures are always stabilized using an antegrade bilateral passage of the nails.

4 Implant removal

Implant removal can be performed after 4 months if consolidation has been confirmed radiologically. The patient can bear weight immediately afterward. The axial alignment and leg length should be evaluated for up to 2 years following the injury.

5 Suggested reading

Schalamon J, Ainödhofer H, Joeris A, et al (2005)
Elastic stable intramedullary nailing (ESIN) in lower leg fractures.
Eur J Trauma; 31:19–23.
Schmittenbecher PP (2000)
Treatment options for fractures of the tibial shaft and ankle in children.
Techn Orthop; 15:38–53.
Till H, Dietz H-G (2002)
Modern trends in the treatment of limb fractures in childhood: shaft fractures of the lower leg.
Kinder- und Jugendmedizin; 2:236–238.
Wiss DA, Segal D, Gumbs V L, et al (1986)
Flexible medullary nailing of tibial shaft fractures.
J Trauma; 26 (12):1106–1112.

6.2 Tibial and fibular midshaft fracture, oblique (42-D/5.1)

1 Case description

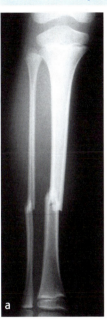
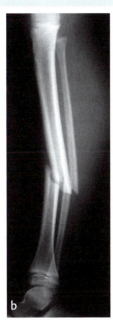

A 9-year-old boy sustained an injury to his right leg when he fell off his bicycle. He presented to the emergency room. X-rays revealed the presence of an oblique fracture of the midshaft of his right tibia and fibula (Fig 6.2-1). There was also significant soft-tissue injury in the distal third of the leg which would have made immobilizing the fracture difficult with a cast alone.

Fig 6.2-1a–b AP and lateral x-rays demonstrating oblique fractures of the midshaft of both the tibia and the fibula. While there was only minimal shortening, the recurvature of both fractures was felt to be unacceptable.

2 Surgical approach

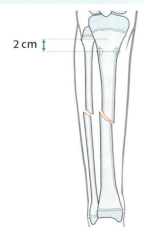

Skin incisions
Symmetrical skin incisions of 2 cm in length are made at the same level on the medial and lateral sides of the tibial tuberosity (Fig 6.2-2). To provide sufficient room to insert and advance the nail antegrade, the incisions must extend from the planned entry site. The subcutaneous tissue is dissected until the dissection instrument is in contact with the cortex of the proximal metaphysis. In performing the dissection, the skin should be incised sufficiently to provide adequate soft-tissue coverage of the cut nail ends.

Fig 6.2-2 The entrance sites are situated on the proximal medial and lateral metaphyseal cortices 2 cm distal to the tibial tubercle.

6 Tibia

2 Surgical approach   (cont)

Entrance sites
The cortex is perforated with an awl or drill. The penetrating instrument is first directed at an angle of 90°. After the cortex has been perforated, the drilling is then continued at an angle of 60° (Fig 6.2-3). It must be remembered that the medullary cavity of the proximal tibial metaphysis has a wide trapezoidal form. This requires that the insertion angle be less steep than with the routine method in the other bones to assure that the nails come into contact with the opposite cortex.

Antegrade insertion
When inserting the nails into the medullary canal it is important to ensure that the tips are pointing into the medullary canal (Fig 6.2-4). As already mentioned, the insertion angle should be less steep to ensure contact with the opposite cortex. If necessary, pre-contour the nails to a more extreme position. Both nails are initially advanced as far as the fracture site by either back and forth rotations of the handle or by applying gentle hammer blows (Fig 6.2-5).

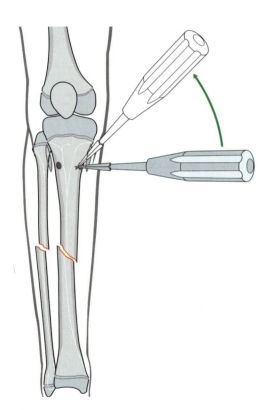
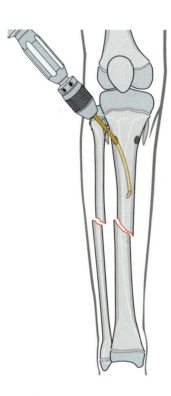
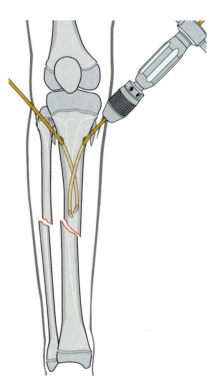

Fig 6.2-3   Drilling of the entry sites.
An awl is used to create the entrance site. It is placed first at 90° and then angled to 60° to the shaft axis to produce an oblique channel in the cortex.

Fig 6.2-4   Nail entry.
The first nail enters the proximal medullary canal. Notice the entrance angle is less steep to ensure contact with the opposite cortex.

Fig 6.2-5   Insertion to the fracture site.
The second nail is inserted and the tips are advanced to the fracture site prior to fracture reduction.

6.2 Tibial and fibular midshaft fracture, oblique (42-D/5.1)

3 Reduction and fixation

Fracture reduction

For the preliminary reduction and fixation, the nail that should be advanced first, is the one that will most easily engage the distal fragment at the fracture site. Usually the fracture can be reduced by advancing the tip of this first nail slightly into the distal fragment. Once inside the medullary cavity, the tip can be rotated to align and reduce the fracture. Once satisfactory alignment has been achieved, the first nail is advanced 1–2 cm across the fracture site into the distal part of the medullary cavity (Fig 6.2-6). The image intensifier is usually necessary at this stage. Once in the distal fragment, the tip of the nail must be directed toward the same cortex that contains the entrance site.

Distal insertion

After this first nail is securely seated in the distal fragment, the second nail is then advanced under image intensification into the distal fragment 1–2 cm beyond the fracture line. Prior to final implantation, the nails are preliminarily shortened, taking into account the insertion length still required plus the one centimeter of the nail that will be left protruding. Definitive anchorage of the nails in the metaphysis is accomplished by hammer blows on the inserter or impactor (Fig 6.2-7).

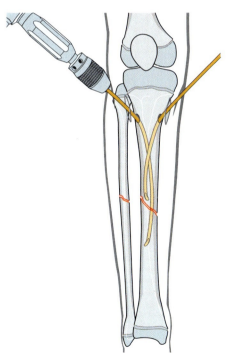

Fig 6.2-6   Fracture reduction.
The tip of the first nail enters the medullary canal of the distal fragment. The nail tip can be rotated to improve the alignment. Note that the tip is directed towards the same cortex as the entrance site.

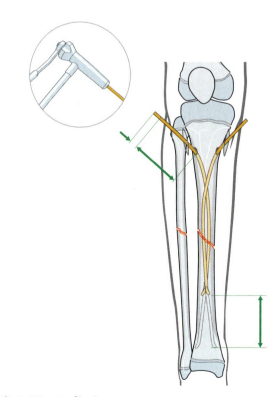

Fig 6.2-7   Preliminary cut.
Prior to the final seating, the nail is first cut, leaving the length of nail equal to the measured distance to be advanced plus the one centimeter of the nail that will be left protruding from the entrance site. The nail tip is then advanced with the hammer to lie just proximal to the distal physis.

6 Tibia

3 Reduction and fixation (cont)

Final seating

Axial compression to fracture fragments is applied to prevent leaving the fragments in distraction. A limited degree of axial correction may be possible at this stage by rotating the nail tips. Preferably, the tips should point in a dorsal (posterior) direction to restore the physiological antecurvature. The beveled impactor is used to advance the nail the final centimeter to position both nail tips immediately proximal to the distal physeal cartilage. If necessary, nail end caps can be applied. The skin is closed over the protruding one centimeter of the nail (Fig 6.2-8).

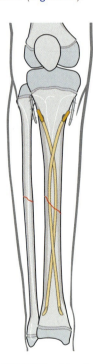

Fig 6.2-8   Final position of nails.
The ends have been cut leaving one centimeter of the nail end exposed. The skin is sutured to embed these exposed tips.

4 Postoperative care and rehabilitation

Postoperative treatment

Immediately postoperatively a radiological check is made which includes the entire lower leg to confirm the adequacy of the overall reduction and alignment (Fig 6.2-9). Following the surgical procedure, the limb can be placed on a cushion or on a foam splint (Fig 6.2-10). Additional immobilization is usually not necessary. Mobility is reestablished with active and passive guided movements of the hip, knee, and ankle joints. Weight bearing depends on individual pain. In some cases, a continuous passive motion splint (CPM) may be utilized.

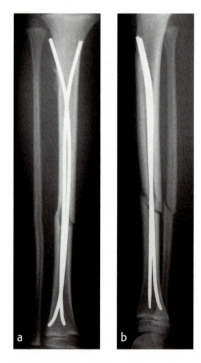

Fig 6.2-9a–b   AP and lateral x-rays taken immediately postoperatively. Notice the tips of both nails are directed posteriorly to maintain the normal antecurvature of the tibia.

6.2 Tibial and fibular midshaft fracture, oblique (42-D/5.1)

4 Postoperative care and rehabilitation (cont)

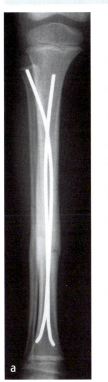
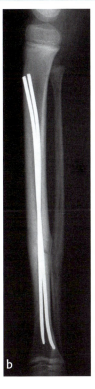

Fig 6.2-10a–b Postoperatively AP and lateral x-rays taken at 6 weeks demonstrate abundant callus.

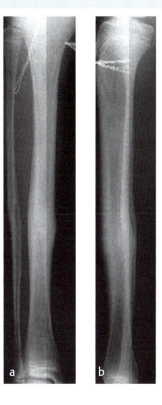

Fig 6.2-11a–b AP and lateral x-rays taken after nail removal (6 months postoperatively).

5 Pitfalls –

Approach
The entrance canal is too steep which will prevent contact between the nail and the opposite cortex.

If the incision is too cranial, there is a risk of injury to the physeal cartilage.

Placing the incision too dorsal or lateral can produce an injury to the peroneal nerve.

In the rare cases where there is severe swelling, closed nailing is not possible.

6 Pearls +

Approach
Less steep insertion of the nail and/or more extreme precontouring of the nail will ensure adequate contact of the nail with the opposite cortex.

Open reduction via small incisions—unless fasciotomy has already been performed to treat compartment syndrome.

5 Pitfalls – (cont)

Approach (cont)
If the nail tips point anteriorly, a fixed recurvature of the tibia may be created.

Rehabilitation

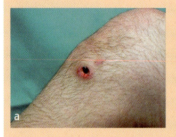
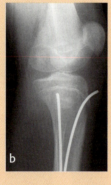

Fig. 6.2-12a–b Excessive protrusion of the nail ends from the cortex of the proximal fragment can result in irritation of the soft tissue with the risk of skin perforation.

6 Pearls + (cont)

Approach (cont)
The nail tips must be oriented in a posterior direction prior to their definitive anchorage in the distal fragment to create normal shape of the tibia.

Rehabilitation
It is necessary to perform shortening as a second stage. It is unwise to leave the nails protruding until consolidation, as this may lead to skin erosion and subsequent infection.

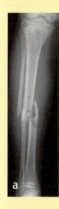
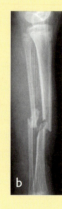
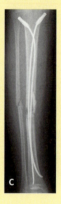
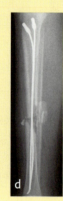

Fig 6.2-13a–d
a–b AP and lateral view of an unstable lower leg fracture of a 12-year-old boy. High risk of shortening.
c–d Longitudinal stability can be achieved by the using end caps. The postoperative x-rays show perfect alignment and correct length.

6.3 Isolated tibial shaft fracture, oblique (42t-D/5.1)

1 Case description

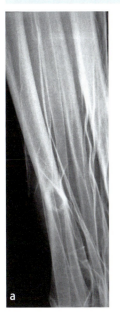
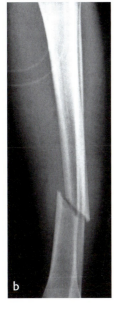

A 12-year-old girl fell while performing in a tumbling event and sustained an injury to her left leg. She was taken immediately to the local children's hospital where x-rays showed an isolated oblique fracture of her left tibial shaft. With the intact fibula, the fragments of the tibia tended to drift into varus alignment. Experience has shown that this angulation cannot be controlled with nonoperative methods alone. It was felt by the treating surgeon that this high-performance athlete required as near anatomic alignment as could be obtained. ESIN was chosen to achieve this end result.

Fig 6.3-1a–b AP and lateral images of the initial x-rays demonstrating both varus and recurvatum angulation of the fragments.

2 Surgical approach

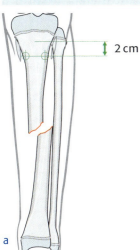
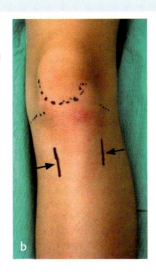

Skin incisions
Symmetrical skin incisions 2 cm in length are made at the same level on the medial and lateral sides of the tibial tuberosity (Fig 6.3-2). To provide sufficient room to insert and advance the nail antegrade, the incisions must extend cranially from the planned entry site. The subcutaneous tissue is dissected until the dissection instrument is in contact with the cortex of the proximal metaphysis. In performing the dissection, the skin should be incised sufficiently to provide adequate soft tissue coverage of the cut nail ends.

Fig. 6.3-2a–b Skin incisions.
a The entrance sites are placed on the proximal medial and lateral metaphyseal cortices 2 cm distal to the tibial tubercle.
b Clinical picture of location of the incisions (arrows).

2 Surgical approach (cont)

Entrance sites
The cortex is perforated with an awl or drill bit. The penetrating instrument is first directed at an angle of 90°. After the cortex has been perforated, the drilling is then continued at an angle of 60° (Fig 6.3-3). It must be remembered that the medullary cavity of the proximal tibial metaphysis is a wide, trapezoidal form. This requires that the insertion angle be less steep than with the routine method in the other bones to ensure that the nails come into contact with the opposite cortex.

Antegrade insertion
When inserting the nails into the medullary canal it is important to ensure that the tips are pointing into the medullary cavity (Fig 6.3-4). As already mentioned, the insertion angle should be less steep to ensure contact with the opposite cortex. If necessary, pre-contour the nails to a more extreme position. Both nails are initially advanced as far as the fracture site by either back and forth rotations of the handle or by applying gentle hammer blows (Fig 6.3-5).

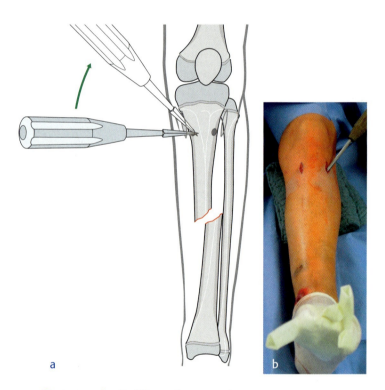
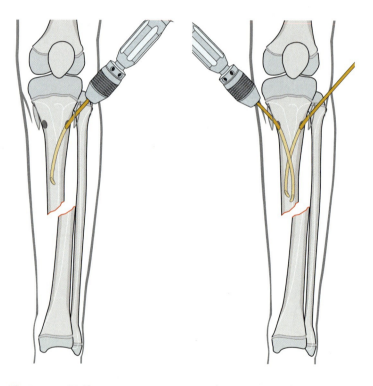

Fig 6.3-3a–b Drilling of entry points.
a   The awl is used to drill the entrance site. It is placed first at 90° and then angled to 60° to the shaft axis to produce an oblique channel in the cortex.
b   Clinical photo demonstrating the final angulation of the awl required to create the entrance site.

Fig 6.3-4 Nail entry.
The first nail enters the proximal medullary canal. Notice the entrance angle is less steep to ensure contact with the opposite cortex.

Fig 6.3-5 Advancement to the fracture site. The second nail is inserted and the tips are advanced to the fracture site prior to fracture reduction.

6.3 Isolated tibial shaft fracture, oblique (42t-D/5.1)

3 Reduction and fixation

Fracture reduction

For preliminary reduction and fixation the nail that should be advanced first is the one that will most easily engage the distal fragment at the fracture site. Usually the fracture can be reduced by slightly advancing the tip of this first nail into the distal fragment. Once inside the medullary cavity, the tip can be rotated to align and reduce the fracture. Once satisfactory alignment has been achieved, the first nail is advanced 1–2 cm across the fracture site into the distal part of the medullary cavity (Fig 6.3-6). The image intensifier is usually necessary at this stage. Once placed in the distal fragment, the tip of the nail must be directed towards the same cortex that contains the entrance site.

Distal insertion

After this first nail has been securely seated in the distal fragment, the second nail is then advanced under image intensification into the distal fragment 1–2 cm beyond the fracture line. Prior to final implantation, the nails are preliminarily shortened taking into account the insertion length still required plus the one centimeter of the nail that will be left protruding. Definitive anchorage of the nails in the metaphysis is accomplished by using an inserter or impactor (Fig 6.3-7).

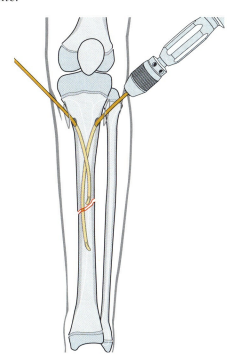

Fig 6.3-6 Fracture reduction.
The tip of the first nail enters the medullary canal of the distal fragment. This nail tip can be rotated to improve the alignment. Note that the tip is directed toward the same cortex as the entrance site.

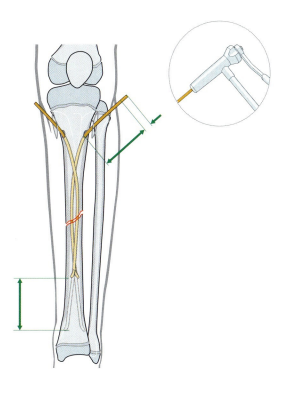

Fig 6.3-7 Preliminary cut.
Prior to final seating, the nail is first cut leaving a length of nail equal to the measured distance to be advanced plus the one centimeter of the nail that will be left protruding from the entrance site. The nail tip is then advanced with the hammer to lie just proximal to the distal physis.

6 Tibia

3 Reduction and fixation (cont)

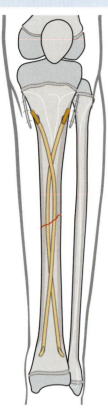

Fig 6.3-8 Final position.
The ends have been cut leaving one centimeter of the nail end exposed. The skin is sutured to engulf these exposed tips.

4 Postoperative care and rehabilitation

Immediately postoperatively, a radiological check is made which includes the entire lower leg to confirm the adequacy of the overall reduction and alignment (Fig 6.3-9). Following the surgical procedure, the limb can be placed on a cushion or on a foam splint. If the fracture fragments have adequate buttressing, no additional immobilization is usually needed. Mobility is re-established with active and passive guided movements of the hip, knee and ankle joints without weight bearing (Fig 6.3-10). In some cases, a continuous passive motion splint (CPM) may be utilized (Fig 6.3-11).

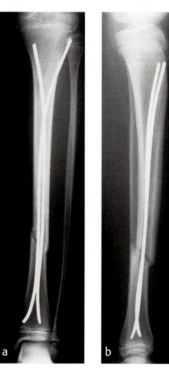

Fig 6.3-9a–b AP and lateral x-rays taken immediately postoperative. Notice that varus and recurvature have been corrected.

6.3 Isolated tibial shaft fracture, oblique (42t-D/5.1)

4 Postoperative care and rehabilitation (cont)

Partial weight bearing is permitted according to the patient's motivation and pain sensation. Often, the child will begin protected weight bearing on day 2 or 3. Subsequent weight-bearing progresses as the child decides.

Full weight-bearing is generally achieved after 3–4 weeks. X-rays taken at 4 weeks often show adequate callus. By 6 months the fracture site has been completely obliterated and remodeled to permit nail removal (Fig 6.3-12).

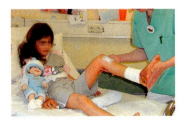

Fig 6.3-10 Active and passive guided movements of the hip, knee, and ankle joints can begin as soon as the patient's pain allows.

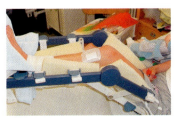

Fig 6.3-11 Postoperative recovery may be enhanced by utilizing continuous passive motion for a short period of time.

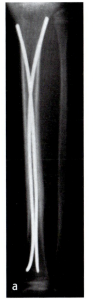

Fig 6.3-12a–b AP and lateral x-rays taken at 7 months postoperative demonstrate full consolidation and early remodeling.

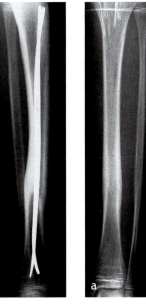

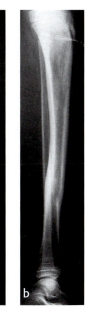

Fig 6.3-13a–b AP and lateral x-rays taken after nail removal (9 months postoperative) show essentially complete remodeling of the fracture site.

5 Pitfalls –

Approach
The entrance canal is too steep which will prevent contact between the nail and the opposite cortex.

If the incision is too cranial, there is a risk of injury to the physeal cartilage.

Placing the incision too posteriorly or laterally can produce an injury to the peroneal nerve.

6 Pearls +

Approach
Less steep insertion of the nail and/or more extreme precontouring of the nail will ensure adequate contact of the nail with the opposite cortex.

5 Pitfalls – (cont)

Reduction and fixation
It is essential to avoid a residual fracture gap. This increases the risk of delayed healing with possible pseudarthrosis formation.

There may be a problem in achieving a satisfactory, closed reduction.

Insufficient axial correction achieved by the implant.

Use of too thin nails will result in insufficient stability. This increases the risk that the nail will bend under load.

If the nail is too thick there may not be enough elasticity which can increase the risk of delayed healing.

If the nails twist like a corkscrew, the internal stability will be lost. This must be avoided.

It is important to avoid alignment in antecurvature.

Rehabilitation
Excessive protrusion of the nail ends from the cortex of the proximal fragment can result in irritation of the soft tissue with a risk of skin perforation.

6 Pearls + (cont)

Reduction and fixation
Apply axial compression at the time of final seating of the nail.

Additive minimal stabilization can be accomplished by means of applying a mini external fixator (one pin per fragment) for a maximum of 3 weeks.

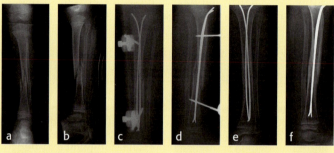

Fig. 6.3-14a–f
a–b Instable lower leg shaft fracture with bending wedge.
c-d ESIN and additional limited external fixation with one pin per fragment for 3 weeks.
e-f Definitive healing and consolidation with ESIN alone.

The nail tips in the distal fragment should be oriented in a posterior direction.

Rehabilitation

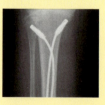

Fig 6.3-15 The nails need to protruding by just 1 cm. Protection of the ends with a nail end cap will often prevent irritation.

6.4 Tibial midshaft fracture, wedge (42t-D/5.2)

1 Case description

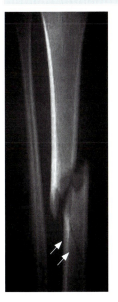

A 10-year-old girl sustained a severe injury to her right leg while skiing. She presented to the emergency room at the local children's hospital with a swollen and painful right leg. Her neurovascular function in the extremity was intact and this appeared to be her only injury. The initial x-rays demonstrated a mid-shaft fracture of the right tibia with a large medially based wedge or butterfly fragment at the fracture site (Fig 6.4-1).

Fig 6.4-1 AP view of the initial x-rays obtained in the emergency room. There is a large medially based wedge fragment (arrows).

2 Surgical approach

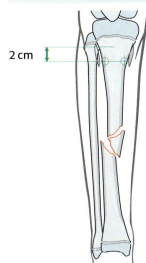

Skin incisions
Symmetrical skin incisions 2 cm in length are made at the same level on the medial and lateral sides of the tibial tuberosity (Fig 6.4-2). To provide sufficient room to insert and advance the nail antegrade, the incisions must extend cranially from the planned entry site. The subcutaneous tissue is dissected until the dissection instrument is in contact with the cortex of the proximal metaphysis. In performing the dissection, the skin should be incised sufficiently to provide adequate soft-tissue coverage of the cut nail ends.

Fig 6.4-2 The entrance sites are placed on the proximal medial and lateral metaphyseal cortices 2 cm distal to the tibial tubercle.

2 Surgical approach (cont)

Entrance sites
The cortex is perforated with an awl or drill bit. The penetrating instrument is first directed at an angle of 90°. After the cortex has been perforated, the drilling is then continued at an angle of 60° (Fig 6.4-3). It must be remembered that the medullary cavity of the proximal tibial metaphysis is a wide, trapezoidal form. This requires that the insertion angle be less steep than with the routine method in the other bones to ensure that the nails come into contact with the opposite cortex.

Choice of nails
The choice of the correct nail thickness is especially important for these unstable fractures. If the nail is too thin, there may be insufficient stability with the resultant risk that the nail will bend under load. If the nail is too thick, then there is insufficient elasticity which can increase the risk of delayed healing.

Antegrade insertion
When inserting the nails into the medullary canal it is important to ensure that the tips are pointing into the medullary cavity (Fig 6.4-4). As already mentioned, the insertion angle should be less steep to ensure contact with the opposite cortex. If necessary, precontour the nails to a more extreme position. Both nails are initially advanced as far as the fracture site by either back and forth rotations of the handle or by applying gentle hammer blows (Fig 6.4-5).

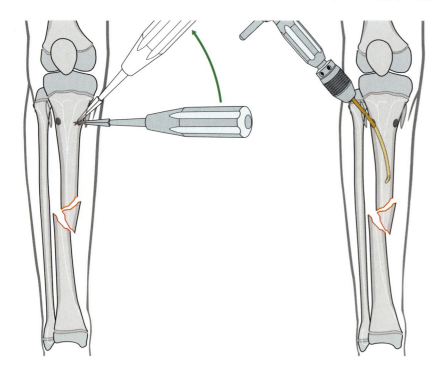
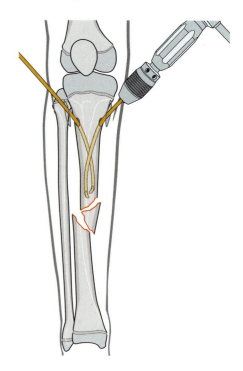

Fig 6.4-3 Drilling of sites.
The awl is used to drill the entrance site. It is placed first at 90° and then angled to 60° to the shaft axis to produce an oblique channel in the cortex.

Fig 6.4-4 Nail entry.
The first nail enters the proximal medullary canal. Notice the entrance angle is less steep to ensure contact with the opposite cortex.

Fig 6.4-5 Insertion to the fracture site. The tips are advanced to the fracture site prior to fracture reduction.

6.4 Tibial midshaft fracture, wedge (42t-D/5.2)

3 Reduction and fixation

Effect of wedge

If the wedge fragment is large, then there is a lack of cortical buttressing on the side of the wedge base. It may be best to initially insert as the first nail the one which will have the maximum bending contour at the apex of the wedge. As a result, an exact reduction may be more difficult due to this instability at the fracture site. Directing the nail can be problematic with this fracture pattern.

Fracture reduction

For preliminary reduction and fixation the nail that should be advanced first is the one that will most easily engage the distal fragment at the fracture site. Usually the fracture can be reduced by advancing the tip of this first nail slightly into the distal fragment. Once inside the medullary cavity, the tip can be rotated to align and reduce the fracture. Once satisfactory alignment has been achieved, the first nail is advanced 1–2 cm across the fracture site into the distal part of the medullary cavity (Fig 6.4-6). The image intensifier is usually necessary at this stage. Once in the distal fragment, the tip of the nail must be directed toward the same cortex that contains the entrance site.

Distal insertion

After this first nail is securely in the distal fragment, the second nail is then advanced under image intensification into the distal fragment 1–2 cm beyond the fracture line. However, its tip may have to be rotated by a maximum of 90° in a anterior or posterior direction. After crossing the distal fracture line, the tip must be brought back to its original position by rotation in the opposite direction. Prior to final implantation, the nails are preliminarily shortened, taking into account the insertion length still required plus the one centimeter of the nail that will be left protruding. Definitive anchorage of the nails in the metaphysis is accomplished by hammer blows on the inserter or impactor (Fig 6.4-7).

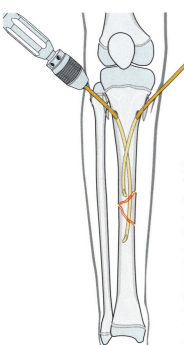

Fig 6.4-6 Fracture reduction. The tip of the first nail enters the medullary canal of the distal fragment. This nail tip can be rotated to improve the alignment. Note that the tip is directed towards the same cortex as the entrance site. In addition, the maximum contour of this nail is located on the side of the apex of the wedge.

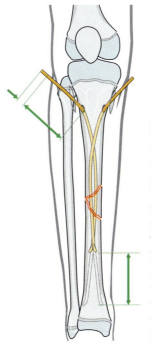

Fig 6.4-7 Preliminary cut. Prior to final seating, the nail is first cut, leaving the length of nail equal to the measured distance to be advanced plus the one centimeter of the nail that will be left protruding from the entrance site. The nail tips are then turned backwards to create the normal alignment of the tibia; otherwise there is cosmetically bad recurvature. The nail tip is then advanced with the hammer to lie just proximal to the distal physis.

6 Tibia

3 Reduction and fixation (cont)

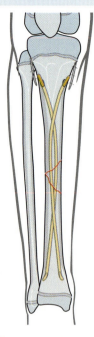

Fig 6.4-8   Final position.
The ends have been cut leaving 1 cm of the nail end exposed. The skin is sutured to cover these exposed tips.

4 Postoperative care and rehabilitation

Immediately postoperatively, a radiological check is made of the entire lower leg to confirm the adequacy of the overall reduction and alignment (Fig 6.4-9). Following the surgical procedure, the limb can be placed on a cushion or on a foam splint. If the fracture fragments have adequate buttressing, no additional immobilization is usually needed. Mobility is re-established with active and passive guided movements of the hip, knee and ankle joints without weight-bearing. In some cases, a continuous passive motion splint (CPM) may be utilized.

Partial weight bearing is permitted according to the patient's motivation and pain sensation. Often, the child will begin protected weight bearing on day 2 or 3. Subsequent weight-bearing progresses as the child decides.

Full weight-bearing is generally achieved after 3–4 weeks. X-rays taken at 4 weeks often show adequate callus (Fig 6.4-10). By 6 months the fracture site has been completely obliterated and remodeled to permit nail removal (Fig 6.4-11).

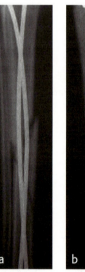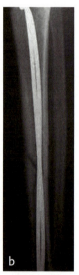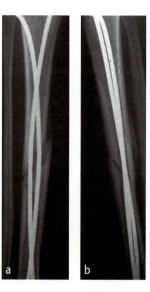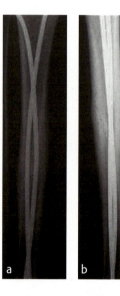

Fig 6.4-9a–b   AP and lateral x-rays taken immediate postoperatively show wide separation of the nail contours at the fracture site which provides maximum stability.

Fig 6.4-10a–b   AP and lateral x-rays taken at 4 weeks demonstrate adequate callus.

Fig 6.4-11a–b   Final healing. AP and lateral x-rays taken prior to nail removal (6 months postoperatively) show complete remodeling of the fracture site.

6.4 Tibial midshaft fracture, wedge (42t-D/5.2)

5 Pitfalls –

Approach
The entrance canal is too steep which will prevent contact between the nail and the opposite cortex.

If the incision is too cranial, there is a risk of injury to the physeal cartilage.

Reduction and fixation
If there is loss of reduction after an attempt at closed reduction with cast immobilization, ESIN stabilization should be undertaken.

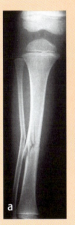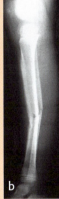

Fig 6.4-12a–b Loss of reduction:
a AP and
b lateral x-rays demonstrating loss of reduction in a fracture treated conservatively. The treatment required a change of management, ie, ESIN stabilization.

If the nail is too thin, there may be insufficient stability which increases the risk that the nail will bend under load.

If the nail is too thick, there may not be enough elasticity which increases the risk of delayed healing or secondary deformity.

6 Pearls +

Approach
Less steep insertion of the nail and/or more extreme pre-contouring of the nail will ensure adequate contact of the nail with the opposite cortex.

Reduction and fixation
If there is any uncertainty about axial stability, the following steps can be taken:
- Keep to short intervals between the follow-up x-rays for the duration of nonoperative treatment.
- Use a thicker implant and/or more extreme precontouring.
- Apply a mini external fixator, whereby only one Schanz screw is inserted at the level of the intersection proximally and/or distally to increase the width of displacement, which will then increase the tension of the nails against the inner cortex (this concept is discussed in chapter 1.1 Biomechanics as "The miss-a-nail technique" and illustrated in Fig 1.1-11).

5 Pitfalls – (cont)

Reduction and fixation (cont)

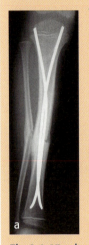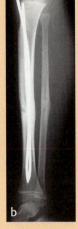

Fig 6.4-13a–b
a AP and
b lateral images of a fracture in which the nails corrected the malalignment.

If the nail twists like a corkscrew, it will not exert adequate tensile force on the internal cortex. This will produce an unstable condition and must be corrected.

Alignment in recurvature must also be avoided.

It is important to avoid a residual fracture gap. This may increase the risk of delayed healing and possible development of a limb length difference.

6 Pearls + (cont)

Reduction and fixation (cont)

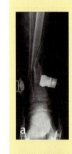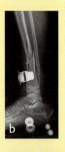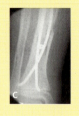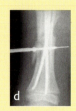

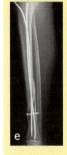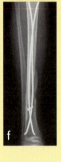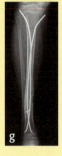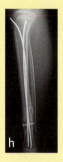

Fig 6.4-14a–f
a–b AP and lateral x-rays of a 14-year-old boy with a multifragmentary lower leg fracture.
c–d Detailed view of screw application; it is recommended that a guide wire is inserted first and then a cannulated screw over the guide wire.
e–f X-rays after 6 weeks show good alignment and correct length.
g–h Good consolidation after 4 months, full weight bearing was allowed after 8 weeks. Nail removal is planned after 6 months postoperatively.

If the corkscrew phenomenon occurs, there must be an immediate substitution of the nails.

The nail ends in the distal fragment should be oriented in a posterior direction.

Apply axial compression when performing the final reduction.

6.4 Tibial midshaft fracture, wedge (42t-D/5.2)

5 Pitfalls – (cont)

Rehabilitation
Excessive protrusion of the nail ends from the cortex of the proximal fragment can lead to irritation of the overlying soft tissue with possible skin perforation.

6 Pearls + (cont)

Rehabilitation
This can be avoided by leaving only one centimeter exposed and protecting the nail ends with a nail end cap.

7 Special indications

7.1 **Pathological humeral shaft fracture (12-D/5.2)** 175

7.2 **Pathological proximal femoral fracture (31-M/3.1–III)** 181

7.3 **Pathological femoral fracture (32-D/5.1)** 187

7.4 **Pathological distal femoral fracture (33-M/3.1)** 193

7.5 **Complex clavicular fractures** 199

7.6 **Subcapital fracture of metacarpal V** 205

7.7 **Radial neck malunion** 211

7.8 **Radial and ulnar malunion** 215

7.9 **Tibial correction osteotomy (unknown unilateral bone malformation)** 219

7 Special indications

1 Pathological fractures

Multiple causes
Pathological fractures in childhood are not rare. The peak incidence occurs between the age 10 and 16 years. The most common causes of these pathological fractures include localized lesions such as benign bone tumors and bone cysts. On rare occasions the tumor may be malignant. In addition, generalized conditions such as osteogenesis imperfecta may predispose the child to fractures following seemingly minor trauma. All these causes are frequently made by pain.

Some of the possible causes include:
- Unicameral bone cysts
- Nonossifying fibromas
- Aneurysmal bone cysts
- Monostotic fibrous dysplasia
- Enchondromatosis
- Osteogenesis imperfecta
- Other rare benign bone dieases

Multiple team approach
Nevertheless, it is of extreme importance to analyze the cause of a pathological fracture. This implies that these fractures should be referred to specialized centers that have a team composed of pediatric surgeons, orthopedists, trauma surgeons, radiologists, and oncologists. These teams should be readily available to evaluate the lesions and formulate specific plans of management.

Original treatment
A multitude of therapies have been described in the literature. One of the most common methods used is the evacuation of the pathological lesion and impaction with autogenous cancellous bone. In many cases supplemental plate osteosynthesis or an external fixator may be needed to provide stability. In addition, some other authors have recommended cannulated screws or steroid injections.

Use of ESIN
Since the introduction of the ESIN technique, it has replaced or superseded most of these previously used procedures. While the ESIN method does not achieve 100% healing rates of the bone lesions, the healing rate is far superior to that for other methods. The bone cysts often do not completely resolve but develop sufficient strength in the surrounding bone so as not to predisposed to a recurrent fracture. Other factors such as localization in the bone, age, and type of pathology may influence the healing rate.

Advantages of ESIN
The ESIN technique provides the following advantages in the treatment of pathological fractures:
- Simple and secure fracture stabilization.
- During the prolonged healing period charateristic of the lesions, additional immobilization is unnecessary.
- Thus, immediate mobilization is possible
- Perforation of the medullary canal leads to the relief of the process, particularly the cysts. This permanent perforation of the medullary canal is accepted also causally for two reasons:
  – the sprout, ie, the immigration of the osteoblasts is facilitated,
  – permanent decompression facilitates bone reconstruction and healing.
- prophylactic stabilization with the possibility for the healing of the process.

7 Special indications

1 Pathological fractures (cont)

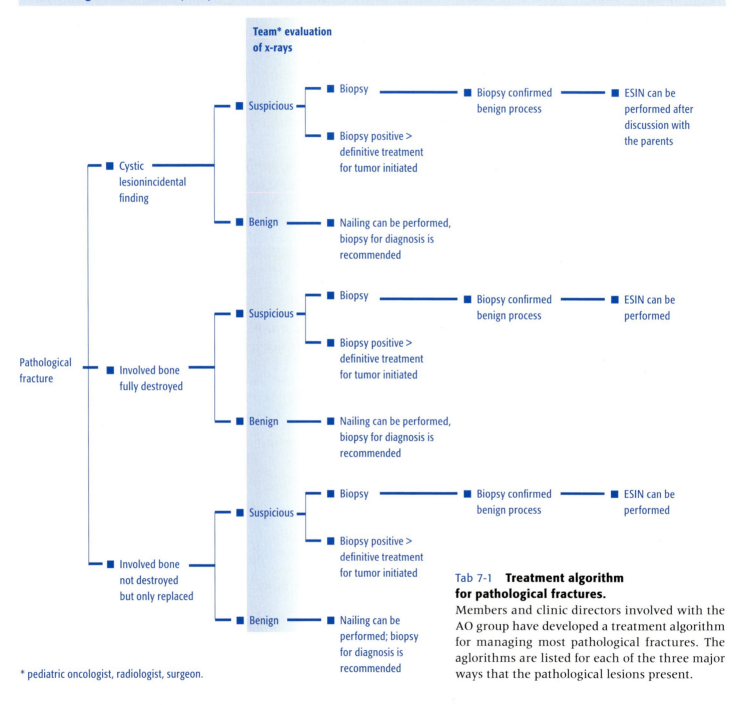

Tab 7-1 **Treatment algorithm for pathological fractures.**
Members and clinic directors involved with the AO group have developed a treatment algorithm for managing most pathological fractures. The aglorithms are listed for each of the three major ways that the pathological lesions present.

* pediatric oncologist, radiologist, surgeon.

7 Special indications

2 Special fractures—clavicle

The vast majority of clavicular fractures can be successfully treated by conservative management. However, cases of nonunion and shortening of the clavicle with poor cosmetic results have been reported even in children.

It is clear that a surgical approach is not commonly indicated and, in some cases, the indications are not strictly defined.

As displaced fractures mainly occur in adolescents it may be necessary to pay special attention to the patient's opinion when weighing up the pros and cons of an operation, especially in girls with fractures of the lateral end of the clavicle.

According to the literature midthird fractures are the most common in children, followed by fractures of the lateral end.

The indications for surgical treatment are as follows:
- Dislocation with potential skin perforation
- Shortening and/or instability of the shoulder
- Possible prolonged morbidity because of impingement of soft tissue
- Open fractures
- Neurovascular compromise
- Risk to mediastinal structures
- Cosmetics

There are indications for the surgical treatment of clavicular fractures, but they are rare and occur mainly in older children. Once surgically treated the results are satisfactory. In our opinion, the best treatment method is in most cases is elastic stable intramedullary nailing.

3 Special fractures—metacarpal

Almost 10% of all fractures in childhood affect the bones of the hand. 72 (21.6%) of the 332 fractures of the hand diagnosed at our clinic were metacarpal fractures, whereby the first and fifth metacarpal bones were affected in the majority of cases.

Although fractures of the metacarpus in children can almost always be treated without surgery, there are specific indications for an operative procedure.

In principle, there are three main issues relevant to surgical reduction:
1. Where is the main deformity and what will be the result of a potential correction procedure?
2. Is there rotation deformity?
3. What will be the effects of a residual deformity in terms of function and cosmesis?

In our opinion, unstable, insufficiently reducible, intraarticular, multiple fractures of the metacarpals, possibly open fractures as well, are indications for internal fixation. The majority can be treated in closed technique.

As for the long bones, the same degree of success can be achieved here with ESIN technique. Especially fine nails or K-wires are used. Since the majority of these fractures are subcapital fractures, the technique is equivalent to that for the reduction and fixation of the radial head.

4 Suggested reading

Capanna R, Campanacci DA, Manfrini M (1996)
Unicameral and aneurysmal bone cysts.
Orthop Clin North Am; 27(3):605–614.

Catier P, Bracq H, Canciani JP, et al (1981)
[The treatment of upper femoral unicameral bone cysts in children by Ender's nailing technique].
Rev Chir Orthop Reparatrice Appar Mot; 67(2):147–149.

Campanacci M, Capanna R, Picci P (1986)
Unicameral and aneurysmal bone cysts.
Clin Orthop Relat Res; (204):25–36.

Imhauser G (1968)
[Management of juvenile bone cysts using intramedullary nailing?].
Z Orthop Ihre Grenzgeb; 105(3):110–111.

Roposch A, Saraph V, Linhart WE (2000)
Flexible intramedullary nailing for the treatment of unicameral bone cysts in long bones.
J Bone Joint Surg Am; 82-A(10): 1447–1453.

Santori F, Ghera S, Castelli V (1988)
Treatment of solitary bone cysts with intramedullary nailing.
Orthopedics; 11(6):873–878.

Wilkins RM (2000) Unicameral bone cysts.
J Am Acad Orthop Surg; 8(4):217–224.

7.1 Pathological humeral shaft fracture (12-D/5.2)

1 Case description

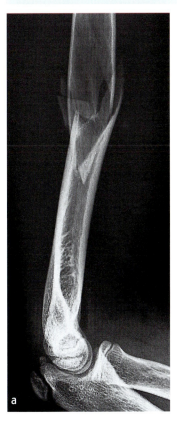
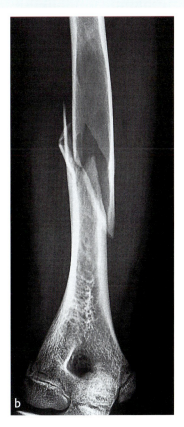

A 14-year-old male was involved in a minor collision with a schoolmate which resulted in injury to his right arm. X-rays of the humerus demonstrated a large lytic lesion in the middiaphysis. In its distal portion, the lesion contained a spiral fracture with an associated free wedge segment. Clinically, this fracture appeared to be unstable.

Fig 7.1-1a–b   Lateral and AP x-rays of the humerus demonstrating a large cystic lesion with a multifragmentary fracture pattern and minimal shortening.

Assessment of the pathology
A team consisting of a pediatric surgeon, pediatric oncologist, and a pediatric radiologist who agreed that the lesion appeared to be benign evaluated these x-rays. There were no malignant changes. The lesion was felt to be consistent with a unicameral bone cyst (see Tab 7-1).

2 Indication

This fracture met the criteria for surgical intervention because:
- It was a very unstable fracture.
- Conservative management would require a long period of immobilization.
- Fractures through these lesions are often slow to heal and become stable.
- Usually, secondary treatment is necessary to resolve the cyst.
- A biopsy may be necessary to confirm the diagnosis of the lesion.

7 Special indications

3 Surgical approach

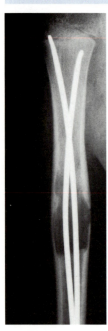

Fig 7.1-2 The ideal fixation with symmetrical bracing of the fracture by the nails is demonstrated in this x-ray.

The standard ESIN technique for diaphyseal and proximal humeral shaft fractures is via a unilateral radial or lateral antegrade approach. This case presents a long fracture zone which is very difficult to stabilize.

In cases such as these the so-called conventional distal retrograde technique with bilateral entrance sites is recommended because it provides better 3-point contact to achieve stability. This is often referred to as the "Tour d'Eiffel" construction.

Retrograde advantages
Another advantage of a bilateral insertion technique is that the nails are much easier to manipulate, which lessens the chance of further injury to the thin cortex. The lateral incision is performed in the usual manner.

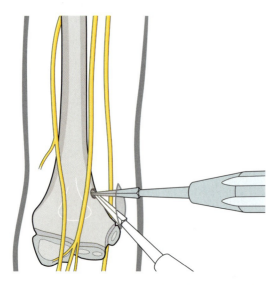

Fig 7.1-3 It is very important to protect the ulnar nerve for the ulnar approach.

Incisions
On the ulnar side, great care must be taken to avoid injury to the ulnar nerve. It is recommended that a large enough incision be made to provide direct visualization of the nerve.

The radial incision starts over the lateral condyle and runs for 3–4 cm proximally.

Distally, the radial aspect of the distal humerus is exposed by blunt dissection down to the periosteum. The exposed periosteum is then incised to facilitate subperiosteal positioning of the hook of the Hohmann retractor anteriorly. This provides direct visualization of the lateral aspect of the distal humerus via a 2×3 cm bone window. The lateral entrance site is created with an awl or drill. It is important to lower the drill to 45° only when the drill is running to prevent breakage of the tip.

7.1 Pathological humeral shaft fracture (12-D/5.2)

3 Surgical approach (cont)

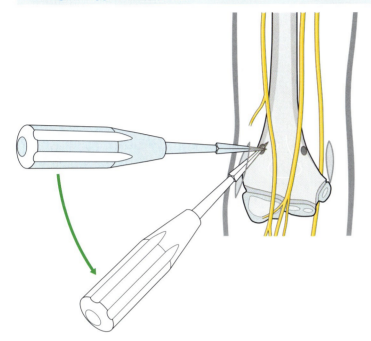

On the ulnar side, a longer incision is utilized. To minimize the risk of delayed injury to the ulnar nerve by the nail this incision is placed in a more anterior location on the arm. Perforation of the ulnar cortex is performed in the same manner as on the lateral aspect. However, because of the narrow aspect of the ulnar supracondylar ridge, extreme care should be used when perforating the cortex.

Fig 7.1-4 The entry point on the lateral side is created as usual.

4 Reduction and fixation

Avoid perforation
The nail is advanced proximally in the usual manner. While the reduction may not be difficult, care needs to be taken when advancing the nail to avoid creating a secondary fracture. Prebending the nail so that the tip does not perforate the bone is recommended.

Nail insertion
The nail is advanced 2–3 cm proximally beyond the fracture zone to insure good stability. Introduce a similar prebent nail on the ulnar side in the same manner. Again, the nail must be advanced very carefully past the fracture zone.

Final sealing
Once the nail has advanced a sufficient distance into the proximal fragment, the nail is cut outside the bone. The remaining distance to the proximal metaphysis must be considered in determining where to cut the nail. It is best to leave about one centimeter protruding from the bone when the nail is finally seated.

The final position of the nail is achieved by the use of the beveled tamp.

Biopsy at the stabilization
Because the nails will most likely remain in the bone for a long time, the tips should be placed very close to the bone. Once adequate stabilization has been achieved, a small incisional biopsy is performed.

| 7 | Special indications |

4 Reduction and fixation   (cont)

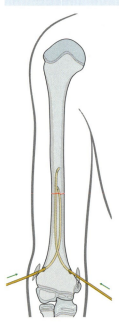

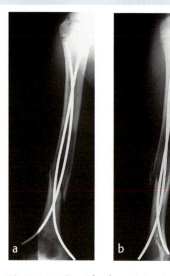

Fig 7.1-5 Nail insertion. Both nails are very carefully advanced past the fracture zone. The arrows demonstrate direction of passage in retrograde technique.

Fig 7.1-6a–b Ideal positioning. AP and lateral x-rays immediate postoperative. The nails were positioned to provide the desired alignment and stabilization.

5 Postoperative care and rehabilitation

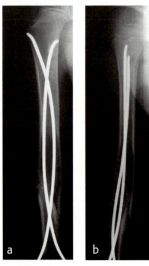
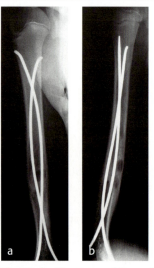

Fig 7.1-7a–b AP and lateral x-rays at 2 months postoperative.

Fig 7.1-8a–b AP and lateral x-rays 1 year postoperative.

Postoperative pain should be managed appropriately. This is usually the normal progression of the postoperative course. The postoperative x-rays should show anatomical reduction and adequate stability to allow early movement.

If after 2 months sufficient callus is visible and the cyst is resolving, the patient may return to normal sports activities.

After 1 year, the cyst should be almost completely healed.

7.1 Pathological humeral shaft fracture (12-D/5.2)

6 Pitfalls −

Approach

The nails have migrated inside the bone because they were cut too short.

In cases involving bone cysts, the nails may remain in the bone for a long time, allowing the ends of the nails to become overgrown with callus.

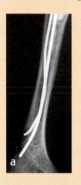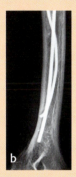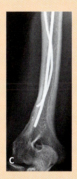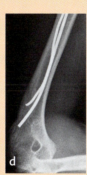

Fig 7.1-9a–d

a–b Nails which stay longer than 2 years in the bone cannot be removed in most cases. At the attempt to remove these nails a great damage to the bone arises and the nails break off.
c–d After one year more the nails are completely overgrown by bone.

The radial or ulnar nerves can be irritated either during nail insertion or by leaving the ulnar nail protruding too much.

Reduction and fixation

Incorrect placement of the nail can produce inadequate stabilization.

If the nails are too short, the cyst may not heal and thus a refracture may occur at the level of the nail tip.

7 Pearls +

Approach

After the first pathological fracture, the fracture may heal with conservative treatment if it is relatively nondisplaced and stable.

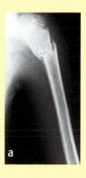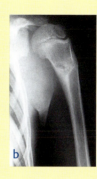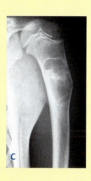

Fig 7.1-10a–c Nonoperative treatment. Since this pathological fracture of the proximal humerus was stable and nondisplaced, it was managed nonoperatively.
a Acute fracture.
b 2 months postfracture.
c 4 months postfracture.

This cyst persisted and continued to grow. It fractured a second time and was again managed conservatively.

With the occurrence of a third fracture, ESIN stabilization was indicated. Subsequent biopsy revealed this lesion to be an aneurysmal bone cyst which may have accounted for the persistence of the lesion.

Reduction and fixation

Lateral radial incision. If the cyst and fracture are proximal, then both nails can be inserted through a single distal lateral incision with separate cortical entrance sites.

Proximal lateral incision. The reduction and fixation are achieved using the conventional monolateral technique via a single proximal lateral incision and separate cortical entrance sites.

6 Pitfalls − (cont)

Reduction and fixation (cont)

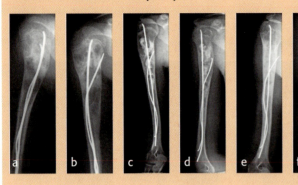

Fig 7.1-11a–f   Refracture.
a–b   Four years previously, this 16-year-old male had undergone ESIN stabilization following a fracture through an aneurysmal bone cyst. Unfortunately, the cyst persisted and a new fracture occurred.
c–d   As part of the treatment it was originally planned to replace both nails. However, only one nail could be removed. As can be seen, there was considerable damage to the cyst wall which required insertion of bone cement for added stability.
e–f   Complete healing of the cyst could be seen 14 months after this combined medical treatment.

Rehabilitation

Despite appropriate treatment the cyst may continue to grow even with the nails remaining in place.

Even after complete healing, the cyst may recur years later.

The cyst may fail to completely resolve.

7 Pearls + (cont)

Rehabilitation
Postoperative recovery usually involves straightforward, painless mobilization. The healing of the fracture and reduction of the cyst should occur within 3 months. Complete resolution of the cyst should be present by 3 years. Bone growth is evidenced by observing an increase in the distance from the tip of the nails to the physis. Unless they are bothersome, the nails need not removed.

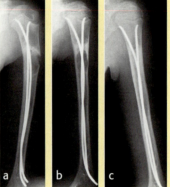

Fig 7.1-12a–c
a   Following this second fracture, ESIN stabilization was performed. A biopsy taken at the time of the stabilization confirmed the diagnosis of an aneurysmal bone cyst.
b   X-ray at 4 months.
c   At 1 year.

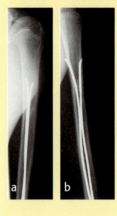

Fig 7.1-13a–b   Complete resolution. AP and lateral x-rays of the completely healed cyst of the patient 3 years post ESIN stabilization. The humerus has continued to remodel and grow. Nail removal is not planned.

7.2 Pathological proximal femoral fracture (31-M/3.1-III)

1 Case description

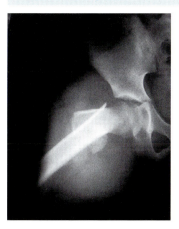

Fig 7.2-1 Initial x-ray showing a displaced fracture through a lytic lesion of the proximal right femur.

A 6-year-old boy fell while playing at his kindergarten. There was the immediate onset of pain, swelling, and deformity in his right thigh. When evaluated in the emergency room, x-rays showed a severe, displaced fracture of the proximal femur (Fig 7.2-1). Initially, it was unclear whether this involved the lateral neck or transtrochanteric region of the femur. The first impression was that this fracture was through a large unicameral bone cyst.

Determination of the pathology

In the first evaluation, because of the large displacement and angulation, it was very difficult to arrive at a clear diagnosis. The case was evaluated by a team composed of a pediatric surgeon, a pediatric oncologist, and a pediatric radiologist. Based upon the absence of any periosteal reaction or signs characteristic of malignancy, this interdisciplinary team determined that the diagnosis was clearly that of unicameral bone cyst. However, because of its localization, an alternative diagnosis was that of an aneurysmal bone cyst.

2 Indication

As there appeared to be no contraindications, it was felt that surgical stabilization was the best method of treatment. The following is a list of the primary indications for the surgical management:
- This appeared to be an extremely unstable fracture.
- It was anticipated that the healing time would be prolonged.
- Because of the instability of the fracture, the immobilization time was predicted to be long if treated conservatively.
- There also needed to be something in the treatment method to stimulate resolution of the primary lesion.

3 Surgical approach

Decision for ESIN

The determination of the appropriate surgical procedure to manage this fracture involves a consideration of various factors. The fracture was very proximal and was surrounded by poor quality bone. This carried the risk of collapse and shortening. Stabilization of the fracture with an angled blade plate or long screws was not able to provide the stability needed.

When these factors were considered, the best solution appeared to be the ESIN technique.

Advantages

The main advantage of ESIN is to provide stability with minimal invasiveness. In addition, it has been the experience of the AO pediatric surgeons group that when ESIN is used, supplemental bone grafting has almost never been required.

3 Surgical approach (cont)

Patient positioning
The child is placed in a free position on the table. A folded sheet wrapped around the groin of the unaffected lower extremity secures the patient to the surgical table (see Fig 5.1-1). This also provides counter traction. The hip must be sufficiently unobstructed to be able to obtain good images with the intensifier. It is imperative to have free rotation of the leg. Preoperatively, the clinical rotation of the nonfractured side must be measured and documented. In some patients, it may also be advantageous to surgically prepare both legs to provide a better clinical evaluation.

Three-nail configuration
Instead of the normal two nails, three nails are used with this fracture pattern. This extra nail, when used appropriately, provides the necessary support for this fracture. The short proximal fragment is supported like a ball on three fingers. The first nail is anchored in the greater trochanter. The second nail is directed into the cranial aspect of the femoral neck. The third nail is directed towards the physis of the femoral head (Fig 7.2-2).

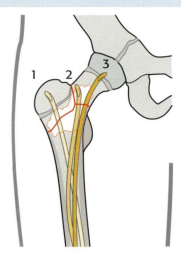

Fig 7.2-2 Three-nail fixation.
A schematic drawing demonstrating the ideal position of the tips of the three nails in the proximal femur. The two laterally inserted nails are advanced to the superior neck and greater trochanter. The third nail is inserted medially to enter the center of the femoral neck.

Medial-lateral entrance sites
To obtain the desired stability, the three nails must be inserted from two separate lateral entrance sites and a single medial entrance site. The lateral incision should be a little longer than normal. Each of the nails is advanced as for the normal retrograde nailing technique.

4 Reduction and fixation

General considerations
The reduction of such proximal fractures is not as difficult as it would initially appear.
It is important to accurately pre-contour the nails, especially in the portion that will ultimately lie within the fracture zone. Continuous traction on the extremity is advisable because of the unstable nature of the fracture.

7.2 Pathological proximal femoral fracture (31-M/3.1-III)

4 Reduction and fixation (cont)

Lateral entrance sites
The lateral incision should be a little longer than usual because of the need to adequately split the fascia lata and provide separate entrance sites. The first nail is inserted following perforation of the lateral cortex at the usual entry point for retrograde nailing. This nail (1) is then advanced to the fracture zone. At this point, the tip is then rotated towards the greater trochanter. It is then driven into the substance of the greater trochanter to obtain preliminary fixation (Fig 7.2-3a).

To prevent splitting of the bone, a second lateral entrance site is made 1–2 cm more proximal and 1 cm more anterior. The second precontoured nail (2) is then advanced up to the fracture zone towards the superior aspect of the femoral neck (Fig 7.2-3b). This nail characteristically has two contours (S-shape).

Avoid cortex penetration
Because the lesion is very large, the surgeon must advance these first two nails very carefully so as not to perforate the proximal cortex with the nail. It is essential to check the alignment of the fracture as well as the direction of the nail at all times with the image intensifier when manipulating the nail tip in the fracture zone.

Medial entrance site
An incision is made on the medial side and the cortex is penetrated in the usual manner as for routine retrograde nailing. This well-contoured nail (3) is then advanced proximally to the fracture zone directing it toward the center of the physis (Fig 7.2-3c). With this third nail, it is important to be careful that the nail does not penetrate the cortex at the calcar.

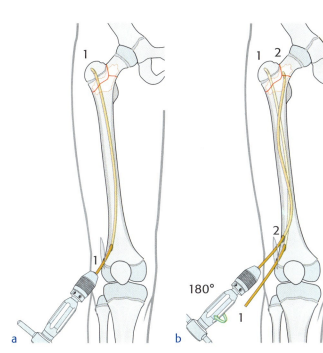
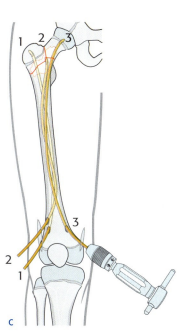

Fig 7.2-3a–d Step-by-step procedure.
a Following fracture reduction, preliminary fixation is achieved by first advancing nail 1 proximaly to the greater trochanter from the first lateral entrance site.
b Nail 2 is advanced proximally to the cyst from a second lateral entrance point. Notice that it has two contours (S-shape).
c Nail 3 is inserted from a medial entrance site to be secured in the femoral neck or head. At this point, the definitive reduction and fixation has been achieved.

4 Reducation and fixation (cont)

Final implantation

Traction is then applied to the extremity and nail #3 is advanced proximally into its definitive position in the femoral neck just short of the physis. It is important at this point to check that the femoral neck is reduced definitively in reference to varus, valgus, and rotational alignment. If necessary, the physis of the proximal femur can be perforated once to achieve better anchorage. Prior to the final seating of the nail 3, it is important to cut the nail to the correct length. The final step in achieving this three nail stability involves advancing nail 2 proximally into the superior femoral neck (Fig 7.2-3d).

Final assessment

Once the three nails have been seated in their final positions, a final evaluation of the stability of the fracture is made. It is also important to check the rotational alignment (Fig 7.2-4)

It is interesting to note that a biopsy of this lesion determined it to be an aneurysmatic bone cyst.

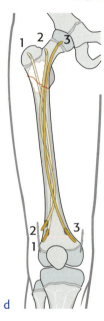

Fig 7.2-3a–d (cont)   Step-by-step procedure.
d   Final implantation. All three nails have been secured in their final positions providing sufficient stability to allow partial weight bearing.

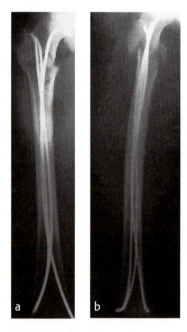

Fig 7.2-4a–b   The postoperative AP and lateral x-rays demonstrate both a good reduction of the fracture and satisfactory positioning of the nails.

7.2 Pathological proximal femoral fracture (31-M/3.1-III)

5 Postoperative care and rehabilitation

Adequate pain management is important.

Initial mobilization
For the first 3 days the child remains in bed. On day 4 mobilization with a physiotherapist is initiated allowing only a toe touch gait. By day 8 the patient can usually be discharged from the hospital having achieved free mobilization on crutches.

Outpatient follow-up
The first out-patient visit is usually at about 6 weeks. The x-rays taken then should demonstrate good healing and callus (Fig 7.2-5). Full weight bearing should be achieved by week 8.

By the next out-patient visit at 3 months, the patient had clinically achieved a free range of motion with equal internal and external rotation (Fig 7.2-6). There was shortening of only 1 cm at the fracture site. X-rays taken at this time demonstrated nearly complete healing and remodeling (Fig 7.2-7). Full sports activities were allowed. Nail removal was performed at 8 months.

Full recovery
By the final visit occurring two years post fracture there was full remodeling with essentially a normal femur on the x-rays (Fig 7.2-8). The leg length discrepancy had disappeared.

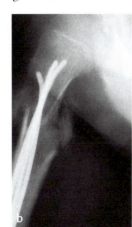

Fig 7.2-5a–b   AP and lateral x-rays after 6 weeks demonstrate good callus formation and signs of early cyst resolution.

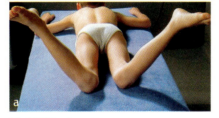

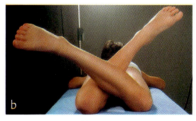

Fig 7.2-6a–b   Clinical recovery. Clinically, at 3 months the patient had a normal range of motion demonstrating equal and (a) normal internal and (b) external rotation.

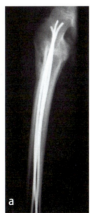

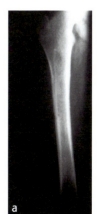

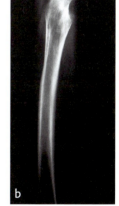

Fig 7.2-7a–b   AP and lateral x-rays after 3 months demonstrating nearly complete healing of the fracture.

Fig 7.2-8a–b   Cyst resolution. AP and lateral x-rays at the last out-patient visit with full remodeling of the fracture and resolution of the cyst.

6 Pitfalls −

Approach
Making the lateral incision too small causes the insertion tools to exert undue pressure on the skin. This can result in skin necrosis and infection.

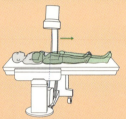

Fig 7.2-9 If the child is positioned improperly, there may not be a clear image with the intensifier.

Failure to measure and record the rotation of the uninjured extremity preoperatively may result in rotational malalignment following stabilization of the fracture.

Reduction and fixation
The child is poorly positioned which may prevent adequate evaluation of the entire fracture.
If care is not taken during the insertion process, the nails can easily penetrate the thin cortex of the cyst.

The nail may leave the fracture zone at the level of the cyst and advance outside the bone into the soft tissues.

The nails are not placed or contoured appropriately in the fracture zone to produce adequate stability.

Rehabilitation
If the ESIN construct is not correct, the stability may be inadequate and additional external immobilization will be required.

The fracture heals adequately but the cyst fails to resolve.

7 Pearls +

Approach
If the reduction is adequate, ESIN can provide good fixation.

It is best to perform the open biopsy first as this allows the reduction of the fracture to be performed under direct vision.

Reduction and fixation

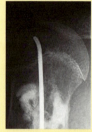

Fig 7.2-10 For pathological fractures in metaphyseal regions, stability can be enhanced by perforating the superior or inferior aspect of the physis of the proximal femur with the tips of the nails. The picture shows a case after chronos inject application in a pathological fracture.

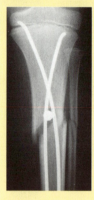

Fig 7-2-11 The inner bracing of the nails can be improved to provide greater stability by the use of a screw. This has been described previously in chapter 1.1 Biomechanics as the so-called "miss-a-nail" technique.

Rehabilitation
While not as stable as ESIN for fractures in normal bone, this construct is sufficiently stable with these pathological fractures to allow immediate mobilization.

As a result, an additional spica cast is not necessary.

7.3 Pathological femoral fracture (32-D/5.1)

1 Case description

Following a rather minimal fall at home, this 3-year-old girl developed sudden onset of pain and swelling in her left thigh. Her x-rays were reported to demonstrate the presence of a nonspecific pathological fracture (Fig 7.3-1). The only treatment that had been performed was to place her in a spica cast for 6 weeks.

According to the original records of her primary treatment, it was stated that the fracture went on to heal. There was no documentation of any follow-up x-rays.

Second episode
Eight months later, she again developed acute pain and swelling in the left thigh. X-rays were reported to demonstrate a large cystic lesion in the proximal left femur (Fig 7.3-2).

The radiographic appearance had changed considerably. It had developed into a large cystic lesion which had penetrated the cortex with a large ossified portion situated outside the intertrochanteric area. Unfortunately, there were no follow-up x-rays after the initial fracture to determine how it had progressed. Because of this situation, the evaluating team felt a biopsy was mandatory. Prior to the biopsy, a full clinical tumor screening examination, including x-rays of the thorax and the appropriate blood tests, was performed.

The biopsy result
Because of the large amount of new bone formation, arriving at the histological diagnosis was very difficult. The final decision was that this represented an atypical aneurysmal bone cyst.

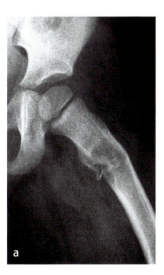
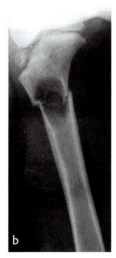
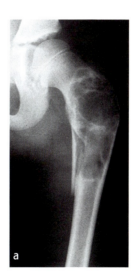
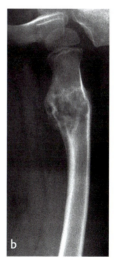

Fig 7.3-1a–b Initial fracture. AP and lateral x-rays of the left proximal femur demonstrate an essentially undisplaced pathological fracture through a cystic lesion. There was no doubt about the benigne nature of the lesion.

Fig 7.3-2a–b Second presentation. AP and lateral prebiopsy x-rays taken 8 months later demonstrate a pathological fracture.

2 Indications

The indications for surgical intervention:
- This represented an extremely unstable fracture. There was a significant risk of a new, even greater fracture resulting in severe loss of bone length.
- It was estimated the healing time of this cyst would be very long.
- Without surgical intervention a long immobilization time was also predicted.
- There needed to be some stimulus to resolve the primary cyst during fracture healing.
- The bulk of the tumor mass would need to be reduced.

3 Surgical approach

It was demonstrated in the previous case (chapter 7.2 Pathological proximal femoral fracture) that the ESIN technique can be used to stabilize pathological fractures of the femur. In this very young child with good healing and remodeling potential, the ESIN technique can be expected to produce good results in both stabilizing the fracture and stimulating the resolution of the cyst.

Three pins required
The proximal location of the fracture zone extending from the base of the neck to the subtrochanteric process dictates that this fracture will require three nails for stabilization (Fig 7.3-3). These nails are inserted retrograde, using two lateral and one medial entrance points (Fig 7.3-4).

A week after the biopsy was performed to establish the diagnosis, the definitive operative procedure was performed. During this interval, the extremity was maintained in traction.

It has been the experience of the AO pediatric surgeons that, when using this technique, supplemental bone grafting to adequately heal the cyst is almost never required.

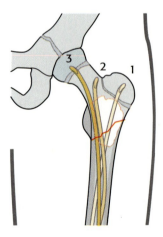

Fig 7.3-3 Three-nail fixation.
Demonstration of the ideal positioning of the three nails, one from medial and two from lateral are necessary to provide maximum stability.

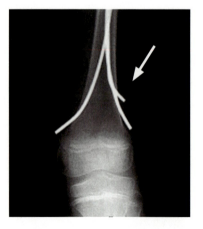

Fig 7.3-4 Entry points.
Location of the two lateral and the medial entry points. The more proximal of the lateral entrance points (arrow) is situated more on the anterior aspect of the femur.

7.3 Pathological femoral fracture (32-D/5.1)

4 Reduction and fixation

Since the exact technique of stabilization has been described in great detail in the previous chapter (see Fig 7.2-3), only a brief outline of the steps will be repeated here (Fig 7.3-5).

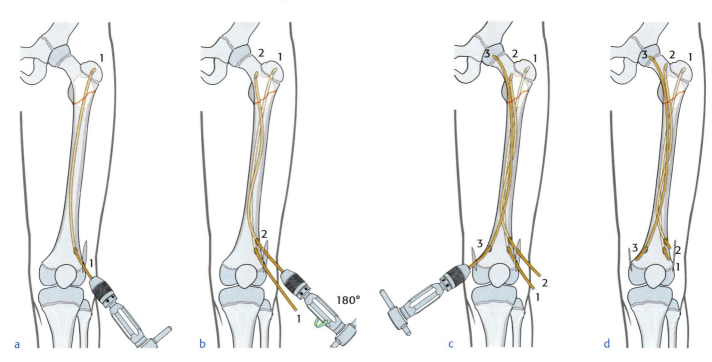

Fig 7.3-5a–d

a Make the lateral incision a little longer than normal to allow for two entrance points. First insert the normally precontoured nail as usual and advance it proximally to secure the tip just below the apophysis of the greater trochanter.

b Next, advance the second nail from a second lateral entrance point so that the tip reaches the proximal aspect of the femoral neck.

c Make the medial incision and insert the third well pre-bent nail from its medial insertion point. The proximal part must be precontoured more than normal because the tip has to advance to the inferior portion of the proximal femoral physis.

d Once the desired alignment has been achieved, advance the nails to their definitive positions and cut the distal ends outside their respective cortices at the distal metaphysis.

4 Reduction and fixation (cont)

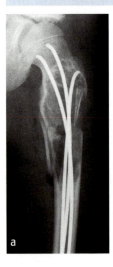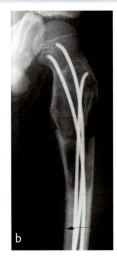

Before terminating the anesthesia, the rotation at the hip is evaluated. The axial stability is assessed by the application of gentle blows against the flexed knee. There should not be any significant change in the axial alignment of the nail when these blows are applied. The final x-ray should demonstrate the ideal placement of the nail tips in the proximal fragment (Fig 7.3-6).

Fig 7.3-6a–b   Final nail implantation.
Postoperative x-rays which demonstrate a satisfactory reduction along with ideal positioning of the three nails.

5 Postoperative care and rehabilitation

Postoperatively, adequate pain management is important. During the first 3 days the child remains in bed. Mobilization is initiated under the close supervision of a physiotherapist from day 4, starting only with normal sitting. A child of this age is too young to mobilize with crutches. In a case such as this, the child is allowed to get out of bed when it is ready. This is usually when they have little or no pain.

Posthospital phase
Hospital discharge usually occurs at around day 9 by which time the child should have free mobilization.

It is usual to have the mother report at 6 weeks that the child is running freely. Therefore, the first out-patient visit need not be until 3 months postoperative by which time healing of both the fracture and cyst should be present (Fig 7.3-7). The child should also be walking without a limp by this time.

Around 1 year after surgery healing should be complete enough to allow removal of the nails (Fig 7.3-8).

Full recovery
A final out-patient visit usually occurs at 2 years after the operation. In addition to complete remodeling seen on the x-rays (Fig 7.3-9), there should be full clinical recovery with normal internal and external rotation of the hips. The leg lengths, likewise, should be equal.

7.3 Pathological femoral fracture (32-D/5.1)

5 Postoperative care and rehabilitation (cont)

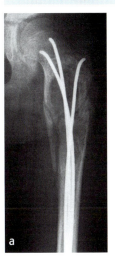 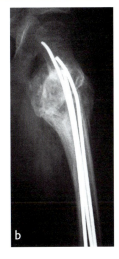 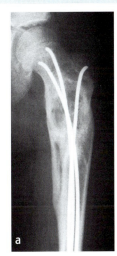 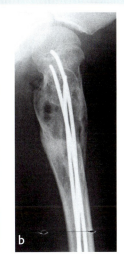 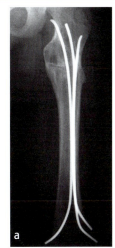 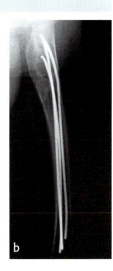

Fig 7.3-7a–b AP and lateral x-rays at 3 months demonstrate good callus formation with complete healing of the cyst.

Fig 7.3-8a–b AP and lateral x-rays taken after 1 year demonstrate complete healing and remodeling.

Fig 7.3-9a–b Final result. AP and lateral x-rays at the final outpatient visit 2 years post-operative. The nails were still in place at the parent's request.

7 Special indications

7.4 Pathological distal femoral fracture (33-M/3.1)

1 Case description

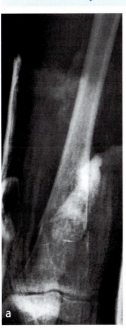
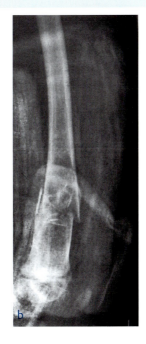

While participating in a soccer match, this 9-year-old boy experienced the immediate onset of intense pain in his right knee after only a slight fall. He was transported by ambulance to the hospital in a plaster cast splint. The clinical examination revealed a painful swollen right knee.
X-rays showed a pathological fracture at the distal metaphysis through an extensive cystic lesion (Fig 7.4-1).

Fig 7.4-1a–b   AP and lateral x-rays of the right femur demonstrate an essentially undisplaced minimal pathological fracture through a cystic lesion in the distal diaphyseal-metaphyseal region.

Assessment of the pathology
These x-rays were evaluated by a team consisting of a pediatric surgeon, pediatric oncologist, and a pediatric radiologist who agreed that the lesion appeared to be benign. There were no malignant changes. The lesion was felt to be consistent with a unicameral bone cyst.

2 Indication

The indications for surgical treatment with ESIN:
- This was an extremely unstable fracture.
- The time for healing of the fracture was predicted to be very long.
- Without surgical stabilization, the extremity would require a prolonged immobilization time.
- There needed to be something in the treatment method that would also stimulate resolution of the cyst along with reduction of the tumoral mass.
- The anticipated long healing time and the shortness of the distal fragment was considered to be a contraindication for external fixation.

Treatment alternatives
Because of the proximity to the physis, the recommended treatment was to reduce and stabilize the fracture utilizing the ESIN technique. An external fixator was considered as an alternative, but it was felt that the ESIN technique provided more advantages and a lower rate of complications.

3 Surgical approach

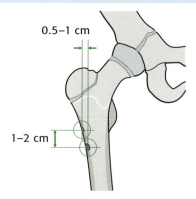

Fig 7.4-2 Proximal entry points.
In the subtrochanteric region, the two anterior-lateral entry points should be separated by 1–2 cm.

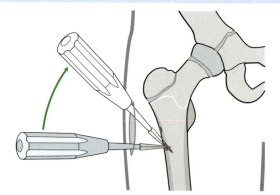

Fig 7.4-3 Skin incision and drilling of entry points.
The proximal skin incision starts just below the greater trochanter and extends distally 3–4 cm to just below the lesser trochanter. It needs to be sufficient to allow enough exposure of the proximal shaft for the two separate entrance sites (small circles). Once engaged, the awl is directed 45° to facilitate antegrade advancement of the nails.

4 Reduction and fixation

The exact technique of antegrade nailing is described in detail under surgical technique in chapter 5.6 Distal femoral fracture. Only the important points of this technique will be repeated here.

The biopsy that was performed prior to ESIN reduction and stabilization confirmed the initial diagnosis of an unicameral bone cyst.

The lateral subtrochanteric incision is made a little longer than normal to allow enough room to be able to have two lateral entry points. Open the medullary canal.

Primary stabilization
First, insert the normally precontoured nail as usual. Advance it distally to the fracture site situated in the cystic zone. Be careful not to perforate or exit through the thin cortex at this level. Use this first nail to stabilize the distal fragment temporarily (Fig 7.4-4a).

Second nail
Once this fragment has been sufficiently stabilized, start with the second nail which has an accentuated precontour in its distal third. Once the second nail is advanced distally to the level of the cyst, rotate it 180° so as to prevent the corkscrew phenomenon (Fig 7.4-4b).

Distal fragment stabilization
Finally, align the distal fragment correctly in both the sagittal and coronal planes.

Once the distal fragment has been properly aligned, both nails can then be hammered into the distal epiphysis (Fig 7.4-4c). Prior to advancing the nails to their final position, they must be measured and cut so that only about 1 cm remains protruding from the lateral cortex of the proximal femur.

In some cases such as the one described here, there may be enough bone in the distal fragment not to need to penetrate the distal physis (Fig 7.4-4d).

7.4 Pathological distal femoral fracture (33-M/3.1)

4 Reduction and fixation   (cont)

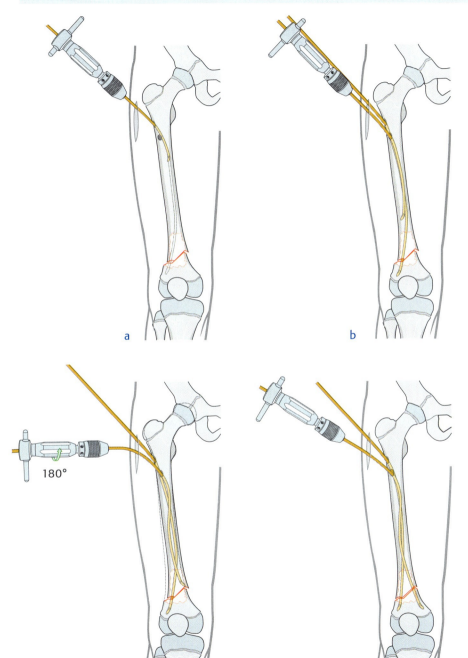

Fig 7.4-4a–f

a   Perform a closed reduction and secure preliminary fixation with the first lateral nail advanced distally from the lateral subtrochanteric region.

b–c   The second lateral nail is advanced distally to the cyst as well. Notice the double contouring (S-shape) of the nail which causes the tip of this second nail to be directed towards the medial condyle.

d   Final tip placement. Once both nails have been advanced to the correctly reduced distal fragment they are driven across the physis into the epiphysis to achieve the final stability into the metaphyseal bone.

4 Reduction and fixation (cont)

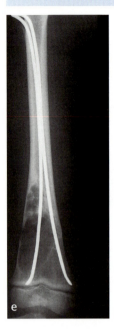
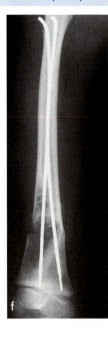

Fig 7.4-4a–f (cont)
e–f Final implantation. AP and lateral x-rays demonstrate a satisfactory reduction with not optimal positioning of the two nails (the first nail should have been more precontoured so that the inner-cortical contact is better). In this case, contrary to the previous figure, sufficient stability was achieved without penetrating the physis.

5 Postoperative care and rehabilitation

Initital mobilization
As in all cases, adequate pain management is important.

Usually the patient remains in bed for the first 2 days.
On day 3 mobilization under the supervision of a physiotherapist is begun with a partial weight-bearing gait.
Since the entry points are proximal, neither the mobility of the knee nor the flexibility of the iliotibial tract are restricted. This enhances the rapidity of the rehabilitation process.

Outpatient follow-up
Discharge from the hospital usually occurs on day 5, having achieved full hip and knee motion. The first out-patient visit usually occurs at 2 months post-operative. If the x-rays taken at that time demonstrate complete healing of the fracture, full sport activity can be permitted.

At the second out-patient visit at 6 months, X-rays should demonstrate complete remodeling and healing of the cyst (Fig 7.4-5).

The healing and remodeling processes should be complete enough at 1 year to permit nail removal (Fig 7.4-6).

Final recovery
At 2 years following the operation, there should be full recovery clinically as manifested by normal internal and external rotation of the hip and equal leg lengths (Fig 7.4-7).

7.4 Pathological distal femoral fracture (33-M/3.1)

5 Postoperative care and rehabilitation (cont)

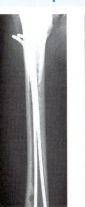
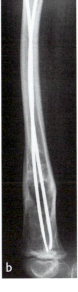

Fig 7.4-5a–b AP and lateral x-rays 6 months postoperatively show nearly complete remodeling and healing of the cyst.

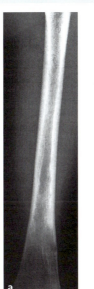
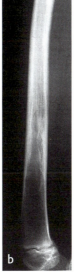

Fig 7.4-6a–b AP and lateral x-rays, following nail removal at 1 year after the primary surgery demonstrate essential bone architecture with the exception of a remnant of the distal canal of the nail.

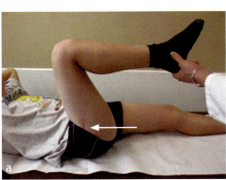
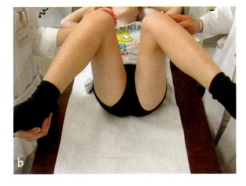
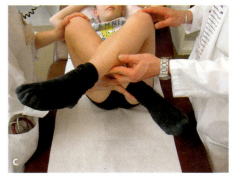
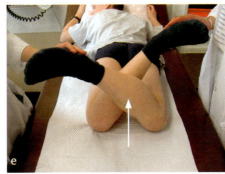

Fig 7.4-7a–e Complete clinical recovery at 2 years. There is
a full hip and knee flexion, the scar at the proximal thigh is visible (arrow).
b Internal and
c external hip rotation with the hips flexed; and
d full internal and
e external hip rotation in extension (arrow).

7 Special indications

7.5 Complex clavicular fractures

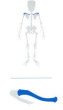

1 Case description

Case 1

A 13-year-old female fell from her bicycle striking her right shoulder directly against the ground. There was immediate onset of pain and swelling at the area of the mid clavicle. The injury x-rays demonstrated midshaft fracture of the clavicle with a rotated intermediary fragment. The clavicle was shortened by 2.5 cm (Fig 7.5-1).

She was initially treated conservatively with a ring or quoit bandage.
She presented 4 days later to the out-patient clinic with severe pain. The skin at the fracture site showed signs of impending skin penetration. There was an increase in the shortening and displacement of the clavicular fragments on the x-rays.

Case 2

A 15-year-old tall female presented 1 year after she had sustained a severely dislocated clavicular fracture. She exhibited an extremely poor cosmetic appearance and experienced pain at the fracture site (Fig 7.5-2).

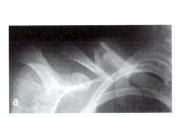 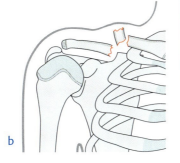 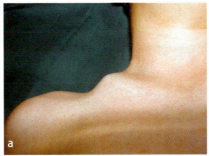 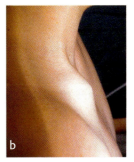

Fig 7.5-1a–b
a X-rays taken at the first clinic visit. The midportion fragments have rotated and shortened.
b Shortening and rotation. Schematic drawing of the shortened clavicular fracture with a rotated intermediary fragment.

Fig 7.5-2a–b Unsightly prominence. AP and lateral views of the right shoulder showing shortening of the shoulder along with a painful prominence from the malunion of the midshaft of the clavicle.

2 Indication

The vast majority of clavicular fractures can be successfully treated by conservative management. However, in some cases of children treated conservatively, there have been reports of nonunion and shortening of the shoulder with instances of poor cosmetic and functional results.

Surgery rarely indicated
Clearly, surgical intervention is rarely indicated. In those cases where surgery is necessary, the indications are not strictly defined. These rare indications, along with the techniques for the operative stabilization of clavicular fractures in the pediatric patient, will be examined in this section.

Primary indication
The primary indications occur in mid-shaft clavicular fractures with severe shortening in the older child. While most of these are simple fractures, there are some with an intermediate fragment which is rotated 90° producing severe shortening. This rotated fragment can also tent the skin predisposing it to perforation.

Permanent deformity
This shortening of the clavicle fails to recover in the older child resulting in an unacceptable asymmetry of the shoulder.

Due to their vast experience with these fractures, the AO pediatric surgeons have determined the following indications for the surgical management of claviclular fractures:
- Severe displacement with potential skin perforation
- Shortening and/or instability of the shoulder
- Possible prolonged morbidity because of impingement on the soft tissue
- Open fractures
- Neurovascular compromise
- Risk to mediastinal structures
- Cosmesis

Two of the surgical indications are examined in the case presentations.

Preoperative planning

Equipment
Since the clavicle is not a complete tubular bone, the so-called medullary cavity is very narrow. This requires the use of small nails such as those with 2.0 mm or 2.5 mm diameters.

(Size of system, instruments, and implants can vary according to anatomy.)

Patient preparation and positioning

Fig 7.5-3 It is important to place the child down on the free end of the operating table. The image intensifier must be situated so that it can be rotated 90° and all portions of the clavicle can be easily visualized.

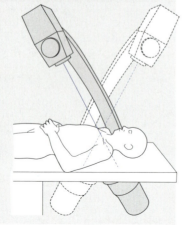

3 Surgical approach

Two primary techniques are available for the stabilization of fractures of the clavicle with ESIN. These two techniques are performed totally percutaneously.

- A percutaneous retrograde technique in which the nails are passed from lateral to medial.
- A percutaneous antegrade technique in which the nails are passed from medial to lateral.

7.5 Complex clavicular fractures

4 Reduction and fixation

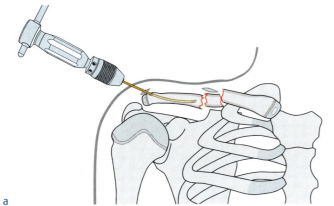

a

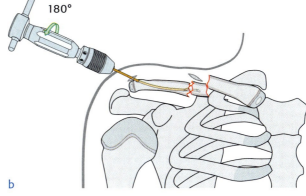

b

Fig 7.5-4a–d Lateral approach.
a   The nail tip is inserted percutaneously into the dorso–lateral cortex of the distal fragment.

b   The nail is advanced retrograde until the tip reaches the fracture surface. At this point the nail must be turned 180° so that the tip can engage the intermediary fragment. Once this fragment is aligned, the nail is then advanced retrograde through this fragment and anchored in the proximal fragment.

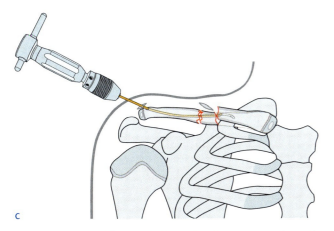

c

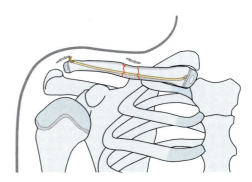

d

c   The nail is advanced through the intermediary fragment into the proximal fragment. In the case presented here, the fragment was rotated through an open incision.

d   Definitive positioning. The nail is rotated until a satisfactory alignment of the clavicle has been achieved.

4 Reduction and fixation (cont)

The lateral approach requires a short incision in the skin prominence over the rotated intermediary fragment (Fig 7.5-4a). Once the fracture is exposed, the blunt end of the nail is inserted through the medullary canal into the distal fragment and then advanced antegrade until it penetrates the dorsal-lateral cortex and skin over the lateral clavicle. The nail is then extracted until the nail tip is even with the edge of the fracture surface of the distal fragment. The intermediary fragment is then rotated through the small original incision so that its fracture surface is in line with that of the distal fragment (Fig 7.5-4b). The tip of the nail is then inserted into the proximal fragment to be advanced retrograde sufficiently to stabilize all three fragments (Fig 7.5-4c).

Because of the impending skin perforation, an open reduction is the procedure of choice.
This involves using the third surgical approach (Fig 7.5-6).

- Make a short skin incision over the fragment.
- The fracture surface of the main distal fragment is exposed.
- After insertion of the blunt end into the medullary canal, a 2.5 mm nail is advanced antegrade into the distal fragment.
- The tip of the nail perforates the distal clavicle proximal–dorsally adjacent to the distal physis.
- The skin is perforated and the nail is extracted.
- The fragments are aligned and the nail is advanced retrograde and anchored in the proximal fragment.
- The nail is given a final rotation to correct alignment of the clavicle.
- Once implanted, the nail is cut to its correct length and anchored definitively.

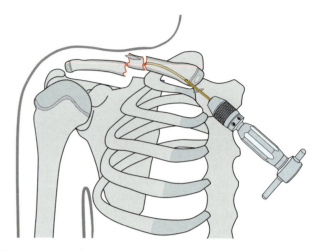

Fig 7.5-5 Medial approach. The nail tip is inserted through a small skin incision medially to perforate the cortex of the medial clavicle. The reduction and advance of the nail in an antegrade direction is similar to that performed in the lateral approach.

Since the indications in children mainly involve fractures with severe shortening and marked rotation of an intermediary fragment, a third approach is suggested (Fig 7.5-6).

7.5 Complex clavicular fractures

4 Reduction and fixation (cont)

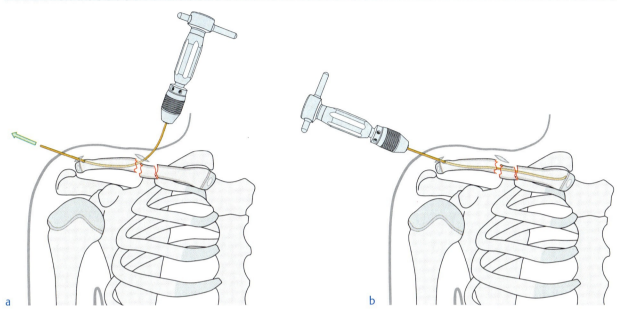

Fig 7.5-6a–b Approach from the fracture site.
a Following careful surgical preparation of the skin, the fracture site is opened through a small incision over the fracture. The blunt end of the nail is then passed antegrade through the distal fragment to emerge through the cortex and skin dorso-laterally in the shoulder. The nail is extracted until the tip is at the level of the fracture site.
b The intermediary fragment is then rotated through the skin incision to align it with the two other fragments. Once the fragments are correctly aligned, the nail tip is advanced retrograde and anchored in the proximal fragment.

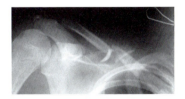

Fig 7.5-7 Initial x-ray. At the initial presentation, a figure-of-eight harness was applied.

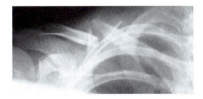

Fig 7.5-8 Development of shortening. The x-ray taken 4 days later at the first out-patient clinic demonstrated significantly increased shortening and rotation of the fragments.

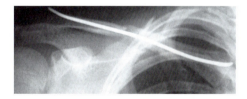

Fig 7.5-9 Postoperative x-ray. Satisfactory alignment was achieved with the x-ray demonstrating exactly the desired position of implantation.

7 Special indications

5 Postoperative care and rehabilitation

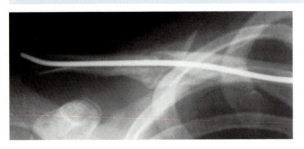

With adequate pain control, these fractures can usually be managed as an outpatient procedure. For more complex fractures, where an extensive procedure was performed, an overnight stay may be necessary for pain control.

Fig 7.5-10 Final recovery. X-ray taken 8 weeks postoperative demonstrates excellent healing and remodeling. Be-cause it was not necessary to take x-rays following nail removal, final x-rays are not available.

6 Pitfalls –

Approach
If the entry point for the antegrade technique is too medial, there is a danger of damage to the sternoclavicular joint.

It may be difficult to open or enter the medullary canal because of the thick cortex.

Reduction and fixation
The medullary canal is too narrow to allow passage of the nails.
A closed reduction cannot be obtained.

Rehabilitation

7 Pearls +

Approach
Avoid creating long unsightly scars as this is particularly important in this anatomical region.

Improperly placed incisions can produce unfavourable cosmetic results.

Reduction and fixation
To prevent proximal migration of the nail into the chest, a small bend is placed in the cut end of the nail as it lies just outside the distal cortex. This bend is then rotated to lie flush against the dorsal cortex.

Rehabilitation
Immediate mobility of the shoulder is possible. It is very important for a child of this age to return to normal activities as soon as possible.

If there is good fixation and realignment, recovery is normally uneventful.

7.6 Subcapital fracture of metacarpal V

1 Case description

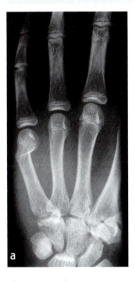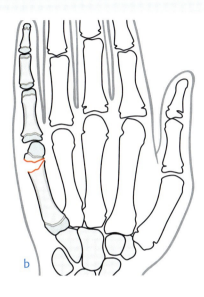

Fig 7.6-1a–b
a Injury x-ray of the hand demonstrating a significantly displaced fracture through the neck of metacarpal V.
b Displacement pattern. Graphic representation of the displacement of the head of metacarpal V.

A 12-year-old boy injured his left hand while participating in a soccer game at school.
The initial x-rays demonstrated a severely displaced Salter-Harris II fracture of the neck of metacarpal V (Fig 7.6-1).

Because of the marked displacement and the age of the patient, there was universal agreement that this fracture required a manipulative reduction. Since these are unstable fractures, this posed the question as to what would be the ideal method of stabilization.
Three possibilities for post-reduction management were considered:
- Closed reduction and plaster cast.
- Closed reduction with K-wire fixation supplemented with a plaster cast.
- Closed reduction and ESIN stabilization eliminating the need for any other immobilization.

2 Indication

As a rule, fractures of the small long bones (metacarpal bones, phalanges of the fingers, metatarsal bones) do not present any complications in the pediatric patient. These fractures usually heal rapidly without problems in those patients up to the age of twelve. However, after that age, the remodeling capacity has ceased and the treatment needs to be more aggressive to achieve a satisfactory outcome. Therefore, fractures even in this area require an anatomical reduction and in many cases surgical stabilization.

The AO pediatric surgeons have found that the best method of management in the present era is to perform a closed reduction coupled with ESIN stabilization. This usually eliminates the need for postoperative immobilization with a plaster cast.
The primary indications for ESIN stabilization in pediatric patients are seen in fractures occurring in:
- Shaft and subcapital areas of metacarpals II and V.
- The thumb.
- The proximal phalanges.
- Metatarsals I and V.
- In rare occasions in the other small long bones.

In adults, this method has become increasingly established as the method of choice.

2 Indication (cont)

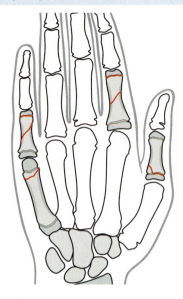

Fig 7.6–2 These fracture patterns in the bones of the hand can be easily stabilized with the ESIN technique.

Preoperative planning

Patient preparation and positioning

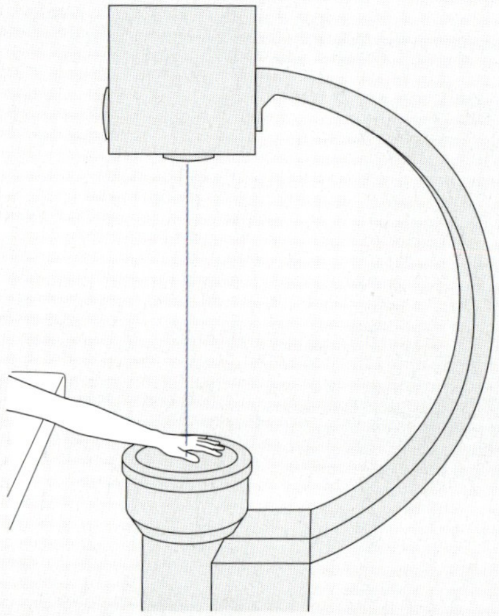

Fig 7.6-3 Image set-up. The correct positioning of the child with the fractured hand resting directly on the receptor surface of the image intensifier. Advantage: better image quality, less radiation.

3 Surgical approach

Normally, the nails are inserted and passed in an antegrade direction. These fractures can also be stabilized with a retrograde technique. The major problem occurs because of the poor soft tissue cover over the end of the nail.

The fracture pattern determines whether it will be best to stabilize with one or two nails. In most cases, one nail is usually sufficient.

This ESIN technique of stabilization for metacarpal subcapital fractures is very similar to that for stabilizing radial head and neck fractures.

Two alterations in the technique can facilitate the implantation of the nails with these fractures:
- First, it is recommended that the operation is performed directly on the receiver of the intensifier (Fig 7.6-3). This improves the quality of the image for these small bones.
- Second, if available, use the magnification program.

7.6 Subcapital fracture of metacarpal V

4 Reduction and fixation

Place the hand directly on the surface of the receiver of the image intensifier.

Entry point
The entry point for the antegrade technique is identified on the dorsum of the proximal-ulnar aspect of metacarpal V, about 5–6 mm distally to the carpal-metacarpal joint (Fig 7.6-4). Confirm the location of the entry point with the intensifier. Perforate the cortex with a small awl or a 2.5 mm K-wire. Cut a 2.0 mm nail 12–15 cm proximal from the tip. Precontour the distal third of the nail. Insert the shortened nail into the medullary canal in the usual manner. The nail is advanced distally to the fracture site (Fig 7.6-5).

Fracture stabilization
At this point, rotate the tip to direct it into the distal fragment (Fig 7.6-6). If the fragment fits well on the nail, advance it another 2–3 mm and rotate the tip 180° to secure the reduction. If necessary, place a finger directly over the fragment to press it into position. At this point, the fragment should be secured in its final position (Fig 7.6-7). The nail is then cut so the end lies with sufficient skin and subcutaneous tissue coverage to avoid later penetration.

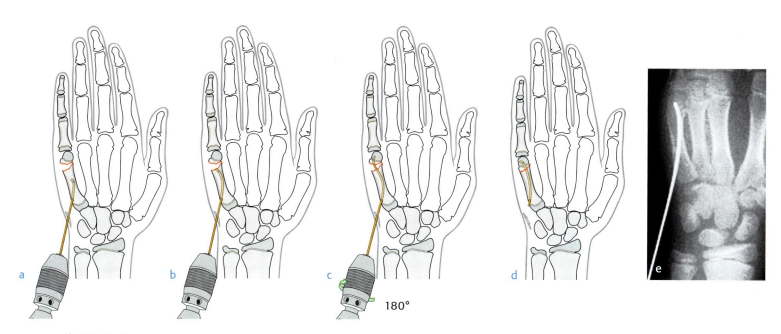

Fig 7.6-4a–e
- a Entrance point. The precontoured nail is inserted into the dorso-ulnar surface of the base of metacarpal V.
- b Antegrade insertion. The nail is advanced distally to the fracture site.
- c Insertion into the head. The nail is then manipulated so that the tip will enter into the center of the neck-head fragment.
- d Reduction maneuver. Once seated in the head, the tip of the nail is rotated to effect a final reduction.
- e Final reduction. X-ray of the final reduction and position of the nail.

5 Rehabilitation

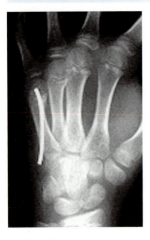

Fig 7.6-5 Final healing.
X-ray demonstrating the location of the nail with callus at the fracture site.

As with all fractures, adequate pain ma-nagement is important.
It is possible to perform this procedure in an outpatient day surgery setting. The degree of pain determines the length of hospital stay.
Additional immobilization and physiotherapy are not usually necessary.
The first outpatient visit and x-rays are performed at 4 weeks. Depending on the mobility of the hand after this examination, participation in school sports activities can begin.
The implant can be removed after 2–3 months, in accordance with the desires and convenience of the parents.
Since no additional x-rays are necessary, x-rays without nails are not available for this case.

6 Pitfalls −

Approach
Because of the thin cortices of the bones and the narrow joint spaces, there is a high risk of perforation of the joint or the cortex (Fig 7.6-6).

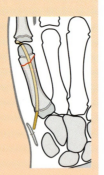

Fig 7.6-6 Joint penetration. The nail is advanced too distally causing the tip to perforate the joint.

7 Pearls +

Approach
Because there is no exposed metal, the infection rate is lower than for the use of cross pins.

7.6 Subcapital fracture of metacarpal V

6 Pitfalls − (cont)

Reduction and fixation

Interposition of a tendon or other adjacent soft tissue may prevent adequate reduction. An inappropriate evaluation of the level of the fracture or direction of nailing can also make it either difficult or impossible to achieve an adequate reduction.

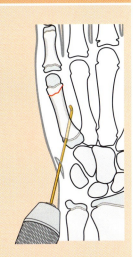

Fig 7.6-7 Cortical penetration. The contra-lateral cortex is perforated with the awl causing the nail to advance outside the bone.

Rehabilitation

Even with the ability to initiate early motion, some of the joints may remain stiff.

7 Pearls + (cont)

Reduction and fixation

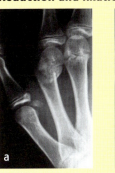
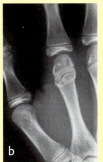
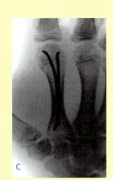
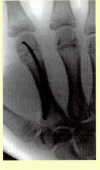
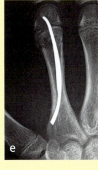
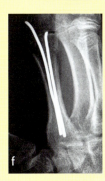

Fig 7.6-8a–f Two-nail stabilization. A Salter-Harris I fracture is stabilized by two nails.

Rehabilitation

Since a postoperative splint or plaster cast is not required, the result is usually a free range of joint motion. This allows a rapid return to normality with regard to participation in school activities.

7 Special indications

7.7 Radial neck malunion

1 Case description

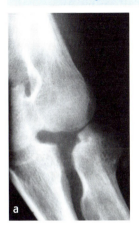
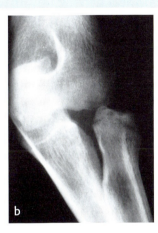

15-year-old female with a 14 month-old skiing injury presented with elbow dislocation and neglected radial neck fracture.

Physiotherapy was started 6 weeks after injury. During the following months she showed persistence of limited elbow motion. Extension/flexion 0°–15°–120°; pronation/supination 20°–0°–40°.

The x-rays at this time showed an angulation of the radial head (Fig 7.7-1). It was recommended to wait, as this type of malunion usually corrects itself in childhood.

Restriction of movement continued for a further 12 months. Therefore a corrective osteotomy was recommended.

Fig 7.7-1a–b   X-rays 14 months after injury; maximal pronation and supination as well as maximal extension.

2 Indication

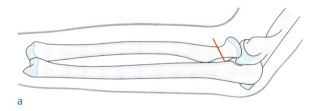
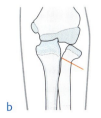

It was obvious that a correction was necessary to treat the severe handicap. Adequate correction must be on the level of the old fracture, meaning intraarticular.

The following options for treatment were discussed:
- A corrective osteotomy and plate fixation which is a complex surgery with a high risk of avascular necrosis of the radial head. On the other hand, a plate fixation also carries the risk of functional problems because of the proximal approach.
- Minimally invasive osteotomy and K-wire fixation with a plaster cast; no functional treatment.
- Treatment based on the concepts of reduction and stabilization of radial neck fractures. With this technique it should also be possible to stabilize a near-head correction osteotomy. This was the method of choice for this case (Fig 7.7-2).

Fig 7.7-2a–b   Planning of the subcapital osteotomy.

7 Special indications

3 Surgical approach

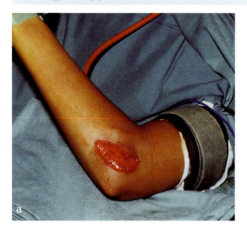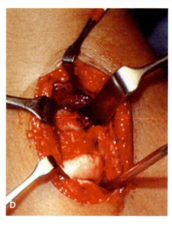

Start with the preparation of the radial neck from a lateral approach. Perform a dorsolateral opening of the radio-humeral joint. Carefully split the annular ligament with a surgical knife. The radial neck can now be seen with the deformation and partial dislocation of the head.

Fig 7.7-3a–b   Radial approach with a 4–5 cm long incision. The capsule is opened exposing the deformed radial neck with subluxation.

4 Reduction and fixation

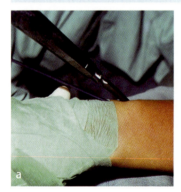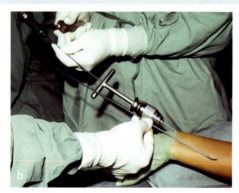

Prepare for distal access at the radius. This is similar to the access used for forearm fractures. Insert the first 2.0 mm nail. Only 2 mm nails are used in this case (Fig 7.7-4).

Fig 7.7-4a–b   Preparation and insertion of the two nails at the distal radius. The outside nail indicates the direction of the nail tip.

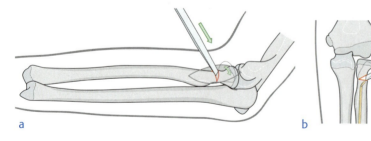

Perform a partial open wedge subcapital neck osteotomy with a chisel or fine saw blade. Good protection of the soft tissue is mandatory. Circulation should not be at risk if the work is done carefully (Fig 7.7-5)

Fig 7.7-5a–b   Schematic drawing of the open wedge osteotomy.

212

7.7 Radial neck malunion

4 Reduction and fixation (cont)

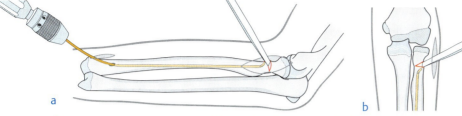

Fig 7.7-6a–b Insertion of the first nail from the distal radial side.

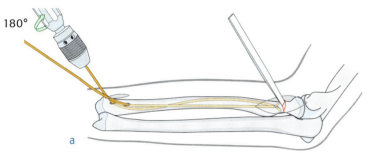

Fig 7.7-7a–b Insertion of the second nail.

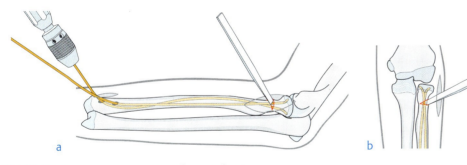

Fig 7.7-8a–b Movement up to the epiphysis.

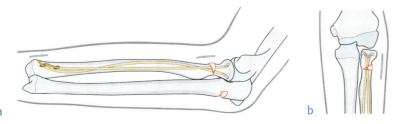

Fig 7.7-9a–b Final fixation in the fragment by both nails.

Open the osteotomy with the chisel, ensuring that the opposite cortex does not break. Now advance the first nail up to the radial head with the tip to the osteotomy side (Fig 7.7-6). Next, advance the second nail up to the osteotomy; the tip is turned 180° in relation to the first one (Fig 7.7-7, Fig 7.7-8).

Cut the ends of the nails and ensure definitive positioning using the impactor (Fig 7.7-9). A single perforation of the growth plate does not matter.

In this case the defect was filled with small bone-block from the ulna. In retrospect this may not have been necessary.

The postoperative x-ray shows a good alignment of the radial head. Intraoperatively the pronation and supination was 60°–0°–60° (Fig 7.7-10).

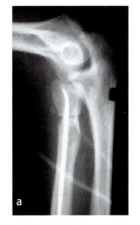
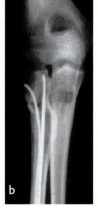

Fig 7.7-10a–b Postoperative x-rays with bone graft in place.

5 Postoperative care and rehabilitation

Because two nails have been used the fragment has been securely stabilized.
The patient stayed in hospital for 4 days. Free range of motion was allowed.
At the first outpatient control after 5 weeks, the patient had no pain, but still limited motion.

Preoperative: Pronation/supination 20°–0°–40°
Intraoperative: Pronation/supination 75°–0°–65°
First control: Pronation/supination 60°–0°–55°

School sport was allowed after 8 weeks. Unproblematic healing was observed.

Nail removal after 8 months. No sign of avascular necrosis was seen at this point (Fig 7.7-11, Fig 7.7.-12). Pronation/supination was 70°–0°–70° comparable to intraoperative range of motion.

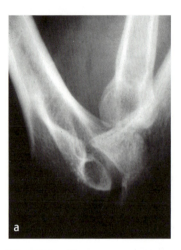
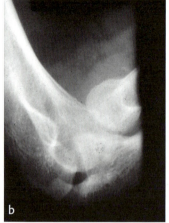
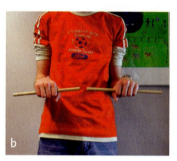

Fig 7.7-12a–b   Clinical situation after nail removal.

Fig 7.7-11a–b   X-rays after nail removal (8 months postoperative) show good alignment and full flexion.

7.8 Radial and ulnar malunion

1 Case description

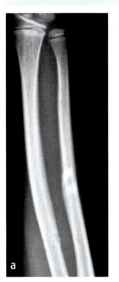
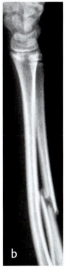
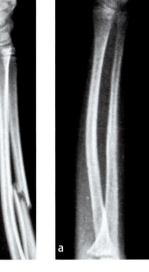
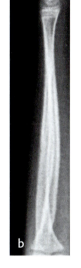

Fig 7.8-1a–b Injury x-ray. Undisplaced fracture of the ulna and severe bowing of the radius.

Fig 7.8-2a–b Situation 10 months after injury.

11-year-old girl fell from a tree onto his right arm. Pain and deformation of the forearm.

The x-ray showed a fracture of the ulna and a bowing of the radius (Fig 7.8-1). The elbow joint, respectively the radial head was unobtrusive. The bowing of the radius could be clearly seen. The fixation was carried out in the plaster cast for 4 weeks.

This resulted in a considerable curvature with restricted pronation and supination (10°–0°– 40°). Ten months after the accident the question of correction arose (Fig 7.8-2).

Considerations:
- The remodeling capacity of forearm shaft fractures is very bad.
- After 10 months the remodeling is complete; the existing malunion will not improve further.
- The child is over 10 years old.
- Functional malunions of the forearm in patients after more than 1–2 years can be corrected anatomically but not functionally.
- Indication is therefore to correct such a functionally bad initial position as quickly as possible.

2 Indication

How can this correction been done? Traditionally, a plate would be used. However, this means a substantial operation and a danger of refracture after plate removal. Plate osteosynthesis is also always associated with large scars.

The treatment option chosen is a minimally invasive procedure with the ESIN method.
- 1–2 cm long incisions at the level of the planned osteotomy.
- Insertion of two nails using a well known technique.
- Functional postoperative management.

215

7 Special indications

2 Indication (cont)

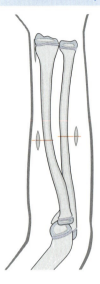

It was planned to perform two osteotomies at the level of the severest angulation over separate short 1–2 cm incisions.
The two nails are inserted from radial distal and ulnar proximal as normal.
Because the ulna is normally straight, it was very difficult to make this correction using a nail.
Therefore, two different minimally invasive methods were combined: ESIN and a small external fixator.

Fig 7.8-3   Planning of the osteotomy.

3 Surgical approach

Standard approach to the distal radius (see chapter 4.7 Displaced distal radial and ulnar diaphyseal-metaphyseal fractures).

4 Reduction and fixation

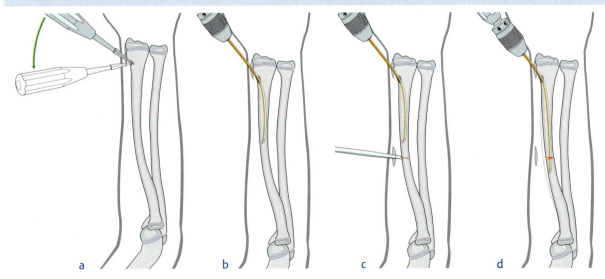

Fig 7.8-4a–d Osteotomy of the radius
a Open the medullary canal with the awl.
b Insert the nail up to the planned osteotomy.
c Make a short skin incision over the planned osteotomy, followed by blunt dissection of the muscles down to the bone. Make an incision of the periosteum and subperiosteal preparation, and insert two small Hohmann retractors. Perform a chisel osteotomy (this heals better, and involves no heat).
d Advance the nail 2–3 cm over the osteotomy.

7.8 Radial and ulnar malunion

4 Reduction and fixation (cont)

Osteotomy of the ulna.

Use the same steps as for the radius (the insertion point is proximal–radial).

Make a skin incision over the planned osteotomy, followed by a blunt dissection of the muscles. Make an incision of the periosteum and put the small Hohmann retractors around the ulna.

Perform a chisel osteotomy.

Now straighten the ulna first, followed by fixation of the pins on a 6 mm connecting rod.

The radial nail can be advanced to proximal now. The nail must be rotated until the radius straightens itself correctly. The pronation and supination must be free.

In this case it became clear that the thin nail which had been used could not correct the deformity sufficiently. Therefore the surgeon changed to a small external fixator to pull out the fragment.

Make four small incisions for the pins (self-drilling, self-tapping 2.5 mm) followed by a blunt dissection down up to the bone.

Using a drill sleeve insert all four selldrill Schanz screws perpendicular to the shaft.

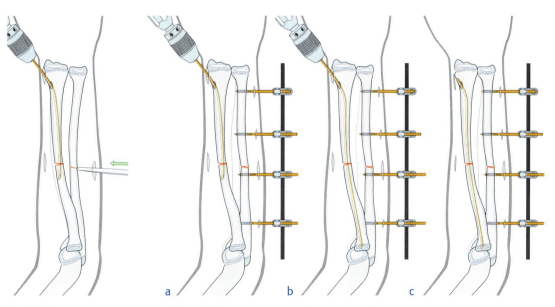

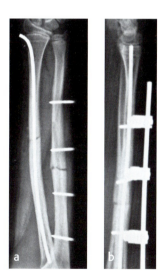

Fig 7.8-5 Osteotomy of the ulna.

Fig 7.8-6a–c Switch to the external fixator and final placement of the radial nail.

Fig 7.8-7a–b Postoperative result.

7 Special indications

5 Postoperative care and rehabilitation

For the first 5 days the patient wore a plaster splint. This was done on the request of the parents in order to cope with pain and anxiety. Free mobility from the beginning would have been preferable.

The external fixator was removed after 5 weeks during outpatient control.

School sport and other sports activities were allowed after 6 weeks. Nail removal after 6 months as a one-day surgery.

After this time full range of motion was achieved (Fig 7.8-8c–d). No further problems were reported.

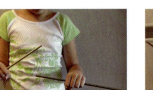
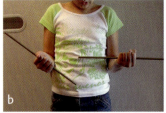
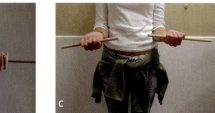
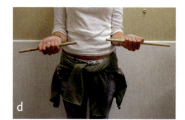

Fig 7.8-8a–d
a–b Clinical situation preoperative;
c–d 3 years postoperative.

6 Pitfalls –

Approach
Changing to an external fixator for the ulna involves three additional small skin incisions.

Reduction and fixation
The nail was not strong enough to reduce the ulna.

Rehabilitation

7 Pearls +

Approach
Osteotomy involves only a small incision. Instead of the one or two long incisions necessary for a plate osteosynthesis.

Reduction and fixation
Stabilization of the osteotomy with two nails would have been simpler, and involved less patient stress.

Rehabilitation
No additional plaster splint, free mobilization from the beginning.

7.9 Tibial correction osteotomy (unknown unilateral bone malformation)

1 Case description

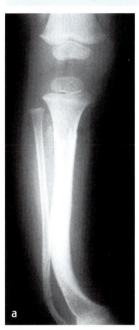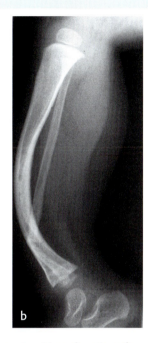

2 1/2-year-old boy, born with a leg length discrepancy of 5 cm on the right leg. This spread out evenly to fifty per cent on the thigh and fifty percent on the lower leg. Both bones were bent, but it was more visible on the lower leg because of less soft tissue.

Extensive examinations revealed no signs of neurofibromatosis, melorheostosis, rachitis, or other diseases. Moreover, the child had a form of dysmorphic syndrome.

The initial opinion was to wait until the child could run. First steps were taken at 14 months. There was no spontaneous improvement or deterioration of the situation.

At age two, walking deteriorated resulting from the malpositioning of the foot.

At this point a possible correction was discussed.

Experience shows that such unknown bone diseases have their own laws. These often contribute to healing problems and nonunions after a surgical intervention.

Fig 7.9-1a–b   X-rays before operation showing the deformity.

2 Indication

In respect to these difficulties, the following procedure was discussed with the parents:
- Carrying out two osteotomies on two levels.
- Stabilization by ESIN, perhaps with a small external fixator for a short time in addition.
- The nail should guarantee inner stability in the case of delayed healing.

219

7 Special indications

3 Surgical approach

Patient in supine position on a radiolucent operating table.

Localization of the osteotomy level with the image intensifier in accordance with preoperative planning. Preparation of the area over the bone with two small separate incisions.

Split the periosteum and put in two Hohmann retractors. Make preparations for both nails and the two entry points. If only one nail can be used, a small external fixator will be applied (rationale: a very narrow medullary cavity is visible on the x-ray).

Before starting with the first osteotomy the insertion of the first nail down to osteotomy level is recommended. Make a proximal, medial skin incision. Perform the bone with the awl.

4 Reduction and fixation

Insert the first prebent nail down to the first osteotomy level. Complete the chisel osteotomy.

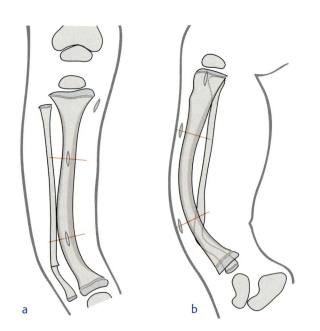

Fig 7.9-2a–b   Planning of the osteotomy levels and approaches to the osteotomy sites and the entry points of the nails.

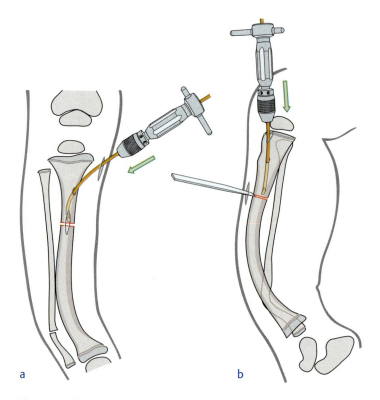

Fig 7.9-3a–b   Preparation of the first osteotomy in AP and lateral view. The first nail (in this case the only nail) is advanced down to this level.

7.9 Tibial correction osteotomy (unknown unilateral bone malformation)

4 Reduction and fixation (cont)

Advance the nail through the osteotomy. Prepare the second osteotomy in the same way as the first one. Complete the chisel osteotomy on the second level. Advance the nail down to the distal fragment. Rotate the nail in such a way that the bend corrects the malalignment. Trim the nails.

In this case, the intramedullary canal was too narrow for the placement of two nails. In this situation the additional use of a small external fixator for rotational stability is recommended.

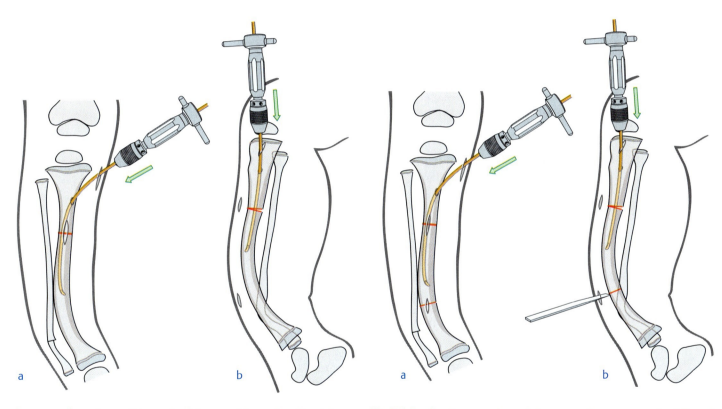

Fig 7.9-4a–b   The nail is pushed forward into the distal fragment.

Fig 7.9-5a–b   Preparation of the second osteotomy in AP and lateral view.

7 Special indications

4 Reduction and fixation   (cont)

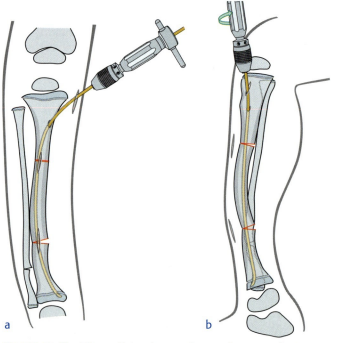

Fig 7.9-6a–b The nail is advanced over the second osteotomy and fixes the distal fragment. By turning the nail, a good alignment of the fragments is achieved.

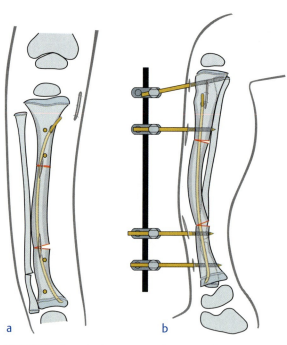

Fig 7.9-7a–b Application of a small external fixator for rotational stability. This fixation is used for 3–4 weeks only. It can be removed when some callus formation is seen.

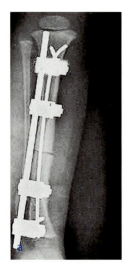
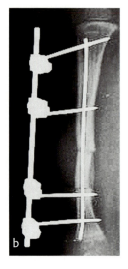

Fig 7.9-8a–b X-rays postoperative corresponding to preoperative planning.

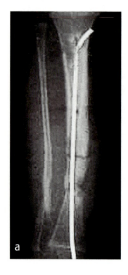
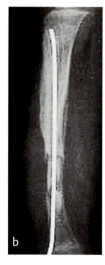

Fig 7.9-9a–b X-rays after removal of the external fixator 8 weeks later. Delayed healing can be seen.

7.9 Tibial correction osteotomy (unknown unilateral bone malformation)

5 Postoperative care and rehabilitation

Despite the two osteotomies, weight bearing was allowed after 2–3 weeks.

Healing had still not led to complete consolidation after three months.

Therefore, the nail was left in place for 1 years.

After nail removal, refracture at the distal level was seen. In the meantime the patient had several café-au-lait spots, and a neurofibromatosis type I was diagnosed.

Our treatment of choice in such a situation is a microvascular fibular transplant. This operation was performed three years after the first surgery.

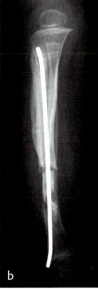
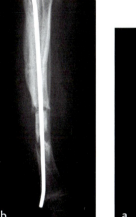
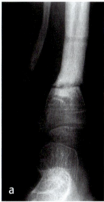
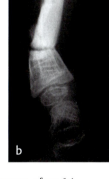
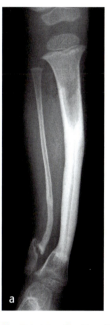
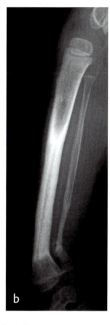

Fig 7.9-10a–b Delayed healing due to neurofibromatosis type I.

Fig 7.9-11a–b Refracture after 14 months exactly on the level where the distal pin of the external fixator was placed 1 year ago.

Fig 7.9-12a–b Rapid healing was achieved with plaster cast immobilization; the malalignment was accepted at this moment.

6 Pitfalls –

Approach
An osteotomy on only one level.
No diagnosis of disease.

Reduction and fixation
Insertion of two nails into the bone was impossible.
The necessity of using an additional external fixator.

Rehabilitation
Delayed healing and consolidation.

7 Pearls +

Approach
Two osteotomies.

Reduction and fixation
The use of an external fixator having realized that the medullary canal was too narrow.
The possibility of using two nails.

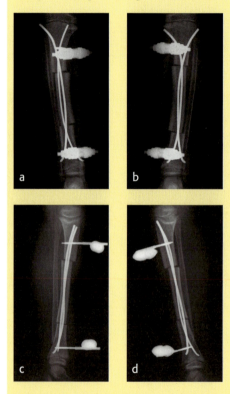

Fig 7.9-13a–d The technique of additional fixation with a small external fixator is demonstrated in this orthopedic case: two-level osteotomies of the tibia and intramedullary fixation with ESIN technique, additional small external fixator to secure the axis and the rotation.
a–b AP view.
c–d Lateral view.

Appendix—AO comprehensive classification of pediatric long bone fractures

1 Introduction

The fracture classification system used in this book has been proposed by the AO Pediatric Expert Group (PAEG) in cooperation with AO Clinical Investigation and Documentation (AOCID) and the International Working-Group for Paediatric Traumatology (IAGKT). This proposal for a comprehensive classification of long bone fractures for children was developed according to a strict validation process [1, 2] and is supported by the AO Classification Supervisory Committee. A more detailed presentation and discussion of this proposal is presented by Slongo et al [3] and further validation studies are ongoing at the time of publication.

The current classification proposal is based on the Müller AO Classification for adults [4] and considers child-specific relevant fracture features (Fig A1-1). The classification process should be conducted based on examination of standard AP and lateral pretreatment x-rays.

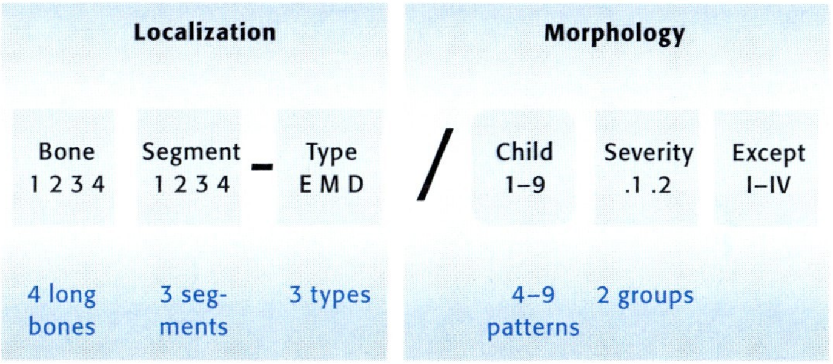

Fig A1-1   Overall structure of the pediatric fracture classification.

2 Fracture, bone, and segment

Following the Müller AO Classification for adults, the bones are similarly coded: 1 = humerus, 2 = radius/ulna, 3 = femur, 4 = tibia/fibula. Except for Monteggia and Galeazzi lesions, when paired bones radius/ulna or tibia/fibula are fractured with the same pattern (see child codes in the next section), a single classification code should be used with the severity code being the worst of the two bones. When a single bone is fractured, a small letter describing that bone (ie, "r", "u", "t", or "f") should be added after the segment code (eg, a code "22u" identifies an isolated diaphyseal fracture of the ulna). When paired bones radius/ulna or tibia/fibula are fractured with different patterns (eg, a complete fracture of the radius and a bowing fracture of the ulna), each bone must be coded separately including the corresponding small letter.

2 Fracture, bone, and segment (cont)

The segments within the bones are coded as 1 = proximal, 2 = diaphyseal, 3 = distal, but their identification differs from adults. For pediatric long bone fractures, the metaphysis is identified by a square whose side has the same length as the widest part of the growth plate in question (Fig A1-2). For the pairs of bones radius/ulna and tibia/fibula, both bones must be included in the square. Consequently, the three segments can be defined as:

    Segment 1: proximal epiphysis and metaphysis (square)
    Segment 2: diaphysis
    Segment 3: distal metaphysis (square) and epiphysis

Malleolar fractures in children are coded as distal tibia fractures (eg, the fracture of the medial malleolus is a typical Salter-Harris III or IV fracture of the distal tibia coded as 43).

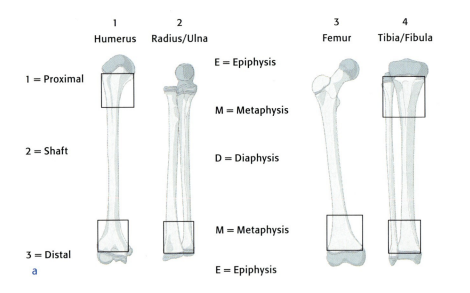
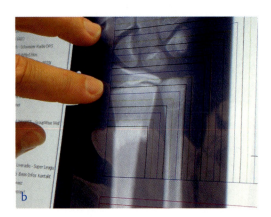

Fig A1-2a–b The metaphysis is identified by a square whose side has the same length as the widest part of the bone physis on the AP radiographic view. For the pairs of bones radius/ulna and tibia/fibula, both bones must be included in the square. The square patterns are copied onto a transparency sheet and applied over the x-ray for more reliable and accurate diagnosis.

Appendix—AO comprehensive classification of pediatric long bone fractures

3 Fracture type

The original severity coding A-B-C used in adults [4] is replaced by a classification of fractures according to diaphysis (D), metaphysis (M), and epiphysis (E). The most common fracture types in children are the shaft fractures (segment 2), and the metaphyseal type (segments 1 and 3). Use of the E-M-D coding identifies intraarticular and extraarticular fractures without ambiguity since epiphyseal fractures are intraarticular fractures by definition. The metaphyseal fractures are identified by the position of the square; the center of the fracture lines must be located in the square (Fig A1-2). This square definition is not applied to the proximal femur where metaphyseal fractures are located between the physis of the head and the intertrochanteric line (see exception code). In applying the square definition, misclassification can occur if the radiological view is not strictly on the AP plane, or the bones are angulated in the frontal plane.

4 Child code

Specific pediatric features (also called "child patterns") are transformed into a "child code". Relevant child patterns are specific to one of the fracture types E, M, or D, and hence grouped accordingly.

The Salter-Harris classification of epiphyseal factures leads to the child codes E/1 to E/4. Other child codes E/5 to E/9 are used to identify Tillaux fractures (E/5), triplane fractures (E/6), intraarticular ligament avulsions (E/7), flake fractures (E/8), and other fractures that may not belong to any of the other categories (E/9) (Fig A1-3).

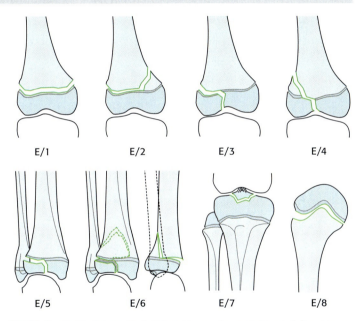

Fig A1-3 Definition of child patterns for epiphyseal fractures.

4 Child code   (cont)

Three child patterns are identified for metaphyseal fractures, ie, the buckle, torus or metaphyseal greenstick fractures (M/2), complete fracture (M/3), and metaphyseal osteoligamentous, musculoligamentous avulsion or only avulsion injuries (M/7) (Fig A1-4).

Child patterns within segment 2 (diaphyseal fractures) are presented in Fig A1-6. They include bowing fractures (D/1), greenstick fractures (D/2), complete transverse fractures (angle <30°= D/4), complete oblique/spiral fractures (angle >30°= D/5), Monteggia lesions (D/6), and Galeazzi lesions (D/7). A 30° angle should be applied to the x-rays for more reliable classification. Similarly, the code /9 should be used for fractures that may not belong to well-defined categories.

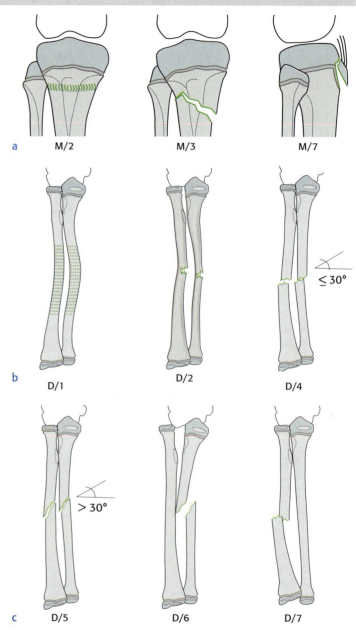

Fig A1-4a–c
a   Patterns in metaphyseal fracture.
b–c   Diaphyseal fracture patterns.

Appendix—AO comprehensive classification of pediatric long bone fractures

5 Fracture severity code

Grading of fracture severity is considered important because of the need to investigate the indications for various methods of osteosynthesis. This code distinguishes between simple (.1), and wedge/complex (partially or totally unstable fracture with 3 or more fragments including a fully separated fragment) (.2).

6 Exceptions and additional codes

Not all pediatric fractures can simply be classified according to the above system, and so a few additional definitions and rules have been agreed upon:
- Fractures of the apophysis are recognized as metaphyseal injuries.
- Transitional fractures with or without a metaphyseal wedge are classified as epiphyseal fractures.
- Intra- and extraarticular ligament avulsions are epiphyseal and metaphyseal injuries, respectively.
- Supracondylar humeral fractures (code 13-M/3; Fig A1-5) are given an additional code regarding the grade of displacement at 4 levels (I to IV) according to von Laer [5]: No displacement (I), displacement in one plane (II), displacement in two planes (III), and displacement in three planes, or no contact between the bone fragments (IV).
- Radial neck fractures (21-M/2 or /3, or 21-E/1 or /2; see Fig A1-6) are given an additional code regarding the axial deviation and level of displacement: no angulation and no displacement (I), angulation with displacement less than half of the bone diameter (II), and angulation with displacement more than half of the bone diameter (III).
- Femoral neck fractures (see Fig A1-7). Epiphysiolysis and epiphysiolysis with a metaphyseal wedge are coded as normal type E epiphyseal Salter/Harris I and II fractures E/1 and E/2. Fractures of the femoral neck are coded as normal type M metaphyseal fractures: mid-cervical (I), basicervical (II), and transtrochanteric (III). The intertrochanteric line delineates the metaphysis.

The full classification code therefore includes 5 or 6 fracture entities depending on the use of an exception code.

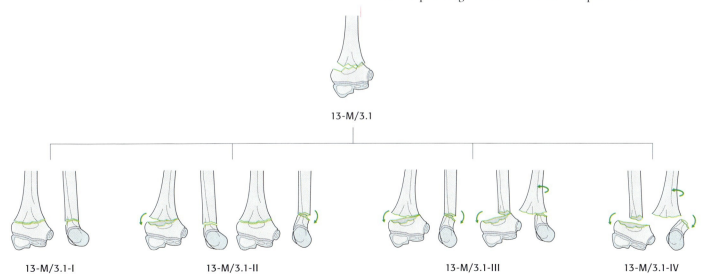

Fig A1-5 Supracondylar humeral fractures.

6 Exceptions and additional codes (cont)

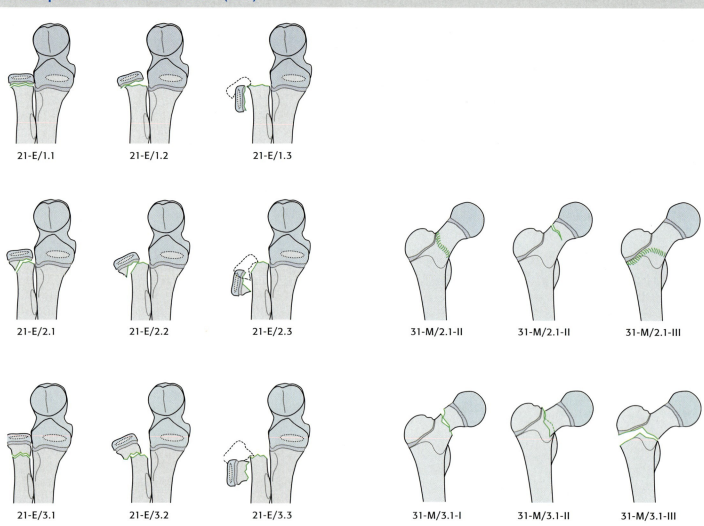

Fig A1-6 Radial neck fractures.

Fig A1-7 Femoral neck fractures.

7 Bibliography

[1] **Audigé L, Hunter J, Weinberg A, et al** (2004)
Development and evaluation process of a paediatric long-bone fracture classification proposal. *European Journal of Trauma*; 248–254.

[2] **Audige L, Bhandari M, Hanson B, et al** (2005)
A Concept for the Validation of Fracture Classifications.
J Orthop Trauma; 19:404–409.

[3] **Slongo T, Audigé L, Schlickewei W, et al** (2006)
Development and validation of the AO pediatric comprehensive classification of long bone fractures by the Pediatric Expert Group of the AO Foundation in collaboration with AO Clinical Investigation and Documentation and the International Association for Pediatric Traumatology.
J Pediatr Orthop; 26:43–49.

[4] **Müller M, Nazarian S** (1990)
The comprehensive classification for fractures of long bones.
Berlin Heidelberg New York: Springer Verlag.

[5] **von Laer L** (2001)
Fractures and dislocations during growth.
Stuttgart New York: Georg Thieme Verlag.

How to use the DVD

DVD

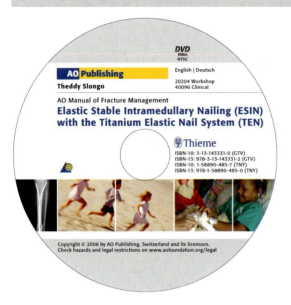

This DVD is an integral part of the book. It provides clinical videos and animations which, combined with the book itself, make the instructive content easier to understand.

Navigation

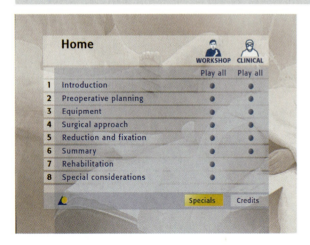

DVD start-up screen: the disc is clearly structured with options for workshop and clinical reality.

The DVD's main menu will show which workshop subject is complemented by a clinical video. The video may then be run by simply selecting it in the menu.

Content

Workshop
Demonstration of the standard surgical technique for elastic stable intramedullary nailing (ESIN) with the titanium elastic nail (TEN) presenting both the antegrade and retrograde approaches to femoral shaft fractures.

Also shown:
- Properties of the nails
- Biomechanics of ESIN
- Instrument set for TEN system

Clinical video
ESIN: 10-year-old child with femoral shaft fracture
Department of Pediatric Surgery
University Children's Hospital Bern, Switzerland

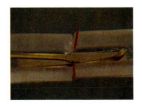
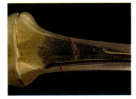
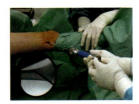

DVD system requirements

DVD player
This DVD can be played on most home DVD players.

Computer
You can view the DVD on your Windows or Macintosh Computer. Any machine that is DVD capable will play AO Teaching Videos. Requires DVD drive, DVD decoder, and DVD player software.